Coronary Heart Disease
A 25-year study in retrospect

CORONARY HEART DISEASE

A 25-year study in retrospect

Menard M. Gertler, M.D.
and Paul Dudley White, M.D.

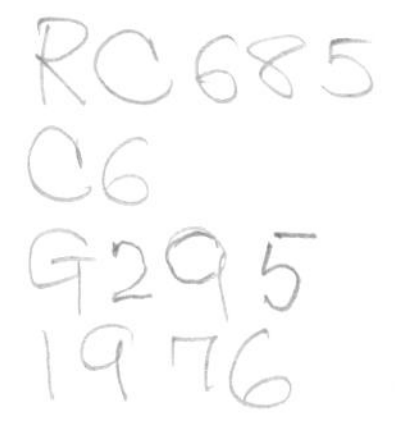

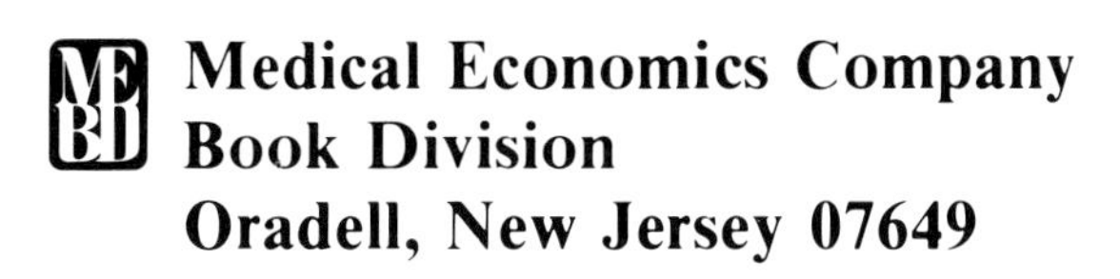
Medical Economics Company
Book Division
Oradell, New Jersey 07649

ISBN 0-87489-093-4

Medical Economics Company
Oradell, New Jersey 07649

Dedication

Dr. Paul Dudley White died October 31, 1973. This was his last major work—the follow-up of the original monograph he had looked forward to viewing "20 years hence." He often referred to the first monograph as a modern classic and hoped it would have an impact on the management of coronary heart disease. The present national and international studies fulfill this hope.

Dr. White was a remarkable human being. He encompassed all those qualities of excellence about which poets and scribes write. His remarkable sense of humor, his sensitivity to human suffering, and his motivation to learn more about the "modern epidemic" were an inspiration to all of us who had the privilege of knowing and working with him.

Therefore, it is fitting that this monograph be dedicated to the memory of Dr. Paul Dudley White.

Contents

Preface

Thirty years ago, a group of medical investigators embarked on a pioneer study of 100 patients with coronary heart disease. The group consisted of Menard M. Gertler, Paul Dudley White, E. F. Bland, J. Fertig, S. M. Garn, J. Lerman, S. A. Levine, H. B. Sprague, and N. C. Turner. Our aim was to compare the patients, whose coronary heart disease had begun before age 40, with other individuals of the same age but without heart disease. Comparisons were made on the basis of heredity, somatotype, and important physiological and biochemical findings. The first results were presented in 1949 at meetings of the New York Heart Association and other groups. They began appearing in medical journals by 1951. The material was assembled and published in book form under our editorship in 1954.

That was before the epidemic scope of ischemic heart disease was fully recognized. Thus, in a sense, the book was at once premature and far advanced. Following publication of the several articles that preceded the 1954 monograph, many individual and combined efforts were directed at finding candidates for the disease and instituting preventive therapy to delay and/or forestall the overt event. The impact of the concept in the first monograph has been so great that, since its appearance, the National Institute of Heart and Lung Diseases has launched a massive program to determine the effect of reducing such risk factors as smoking, hypertension, and serum cholesterol on the incidence, prevalence, and morbidity of coronary heart disease.

This volume presents a long-term follow-up of the original coronary and control groups. In addition, it reviews and assesses the status of heart disease research, thereby enabling the reader to interpret the meaning of our results. The review of the literature also demonstrates how other investigators, particularly the Framingham group, have confirmed and/or extended the concepts we first proposed.

The authors are grateful to many individuals who aided them during the follow-up of patients and control subjects and who were instrumental in the completion of the manuscript. We are particularly indebted to Mrs. Elyse Johnson for her tremendous dedication to the project; she did an excellent job in the final collection of data and in the preparation of the manuscript. We are grateful to Miss Margaret Thayer and Dr. Florence Avitabile for their help in tracing our patients and collecting the data. We owe thanks to Dr. Ionel Bandu for his help in examining many of the patients. We must single out our associates James Rosenberger and Russell Koutrouby for their masterful and sensitive interpretation of the statistical data. A debt of gratitude is owed Dr. Howard A. Rusk for his help and constant cooperation.

To the physicians of the coronary and control subjects (too numerous to mention here, but included in the appendix), we extend our deep appreciation. Their assistance in examining patients and control subjects and reporting the data in a form suitable for computer analysis was invaluable.

The authors are deeply indebted to The Commonwealth Fund in New York City for its generous support, without which the follow-up studies and manuscript revision could not have been completed. We thank Harvard University Press for its kind permission to reproduce background material from the original monograph (copyright 1954 by The Commonwealth Fund).

Finally, we call attention to the patients and control subjects who gave their time and effort to help others avoid the "modern epidemic."

I Introduction: The Problem and the Procedure

Coronary heart disease continues to be a major world problem, accounting for 35 per cent of the total deaths that occur in the U.S. alone.[1] This exceeds the number of deaths caused by the next three biggest killers combined—cancer, stroke, and accidents. To be sure, mortality for arteriosclerosis declined by 1.2 per cent between 1967 and 1968, but not before rising at a rate of 11.1 per 100,000 in the preceding decade (1955-1965).[2]

The acknowledged importance of atherosclerosis in the etiology of coronary heart disease prompted early investigators to search for clues to the origin of coronary heart disease. Their findings culminated in the description of a group of parameters, which became known over the next 20 years as "risk factors." Today, these risk factors help identify candidates for the disease *in its covert stage,* thereby enabling the physician to employ methods of interference to delay and/or prevent the disease from reaching the overt stage.

The history of the present study goes back to 1937, when Glendy, Levine, and White published a report comparing 100 coronary heart disease patients under the age of 40 with a group of healthy older people. In the course of their research, the investigators made two important findings: (a) Out of a population with as many females as males, there were 96 males but only four females in the coronary group, and (b) the majority of the patients were husky, or mesomorphic, in build. Another interesting fact was that the healthy older people had had, in their youth, many more infectious diseases (such as diphtheria and typhoid fever) than the coronary patients. Unfortunately, a deeper look into these subjects was cut short by the outbreak of World War II, but the questions that had been raised stayed in the minds of the investigators. This is apparent in the third edition (1944) of Paul Dudley White's *Heart Disease,* in which the author muses, "Why should the robust and apparently most masculine young male be particularly prone to this disease?" Interestingly, Levine in 1929 had already described the male especially subject to coronary thrombosis as being short, thickset, obese, and with thick wrists.

On the basis of these earlier developments and because of the increasingly compelling challenge that coronary disease posed, a new research study of atherosclerosis in young adults was organized as soon as postwar conditions permitted. There were many loose clues; in an effort to make sense of them, the morphological, genetic, athletic, occupational, physiological, clinical, dietary, hormonal, and biochemical aspects of the disease were explored.[3]

Selection of Patients

In selecting patients, an upper age limit was set in the belief that the individual who experienced a coronary occlusion at an early age would show predisposing characteristics to it. The guidelines adopted by Glendy, Levine, and White required that subjects be 40 years or younger at the time of myocardial infarction and less than 50 at the time of examination. The limit was set at 40, rather than 30 or 35, as a matter of practicality in obtaining patients. Although the youngest patient in the series was 24 at the time of his myocardial infarction, the majority (61 out of 97 males) had MIs between 25 and 40.

Patients were accepted for study in the Coronary Research Project only after meeting certain other requirements: They had to be in ambulatory condition; they had to have had a myocardial infarction at least six months earlier; and they had to be free of diabetes mellitus, syphilis, and other serious infections. Additionally, there could be no hypertension at the time of the study (one patient had undergone a successful lumbo-dorsal sympathectomy for previous hypertension). The 100 patients finally accepted into the study were culled from approximately 250 referrals.

Selection of Controls

A general or unmatched control group of 146 males was originally employed for control purposes. Ultimately, however, the experimentally ideal matched-pair technique was adopted to avoid such problems as differences in height and weight between patients and unmatched controls might create. Thus, matches were made on an individual basis, with each matched control closely resembling a coronary patient in age, height, weight, body build, ethnic origin, and occupation. This group of 97 males will be referred to as the matched control group.

Follow-up

Our original study on coronary heart disease was the first of its kind, since it embraced two new and innovative concepts:

1. The use of 100 cases of "pure" coronary heart disease (absence of hypertension, diabetes mellitus, and xanthomatosis) in individuals under the age of 40 at the time of their first episode. This gave us the unique opportunity to observe the natural history of the disease with current medical and secondary prevention techniques. It also enabled us to observe the effects of single and multiple risk factors on the survival period of each propositus. Each risk factor, it was thought, could be assessed in terms of its importance. Depending on the outcome of that assessment, the risk factor would either be used in or eliminated from future studies. The advantages in following a known disease group over a healthy group were apparent: Waiting for development of the disease was shorter, and the factors thought to be predictive could be assessed more accurately.
2. The pursuit of a long-term follow-up of 146 healthy men, making this one of the earliest epidemiological studies ever undertaken. The parameters associated with coronary heart disease were applied to this group, and candidates for the disease were singled out to determine the accuracy of our predictive measures. The character of the group also offered us the opportunity to assess the changing pattern of risk factors to determine their significance in the development of overt coronary heart disease.

Locating the original coronary and control group members as well as their families was a long and difficult process. After a full year of investigation we were able to determine the whereabouts of approximately 99 per cent of both groups, as well as obtain information on the number of deaths that had occurred. In many instances study participants still resided in the same town or city as when the study began in 1947. Changes of address were often furnished by family physicians as well as relatives. Various state agencies and hospitals assisted in the search for missing study participants and their families, but, when these efforts failed, the aid of missing persons bureaus was enlisted. Deaths were verified by city clerks in the respective areas, and hospital and physicians' records as well as death certificates were sought to obtain information on the circumstances surrounding each incident. The families of the coronary victims were extremely helpful in providing this vital data.

Twenty of the 21 coronary patients known to be alive were examined by either their personal physicians or by the authors in Boston or New York. In addition to the routine physical examination, thorough blood studies and electrocardiograms were done to determine the physical status of each coronary patient. All serum lipid analyses were performed in our laboratory. The same procedure was followed for the control group members; of the original 125 participants known to be alive, 115 controls were examined, although one of their number died shortly after being re-examined.

Throughout the course of the follow-up it was impossible to obtain data on every variable for every subject. This was due to the fact that many private physicians performing the examinations did not always report the complete results. In addition, there were some subjects who would not return for a second examination when data were found to be missing. Often patients could not remember details about such things as family history of heart disease and past smoking, drinking, and eating habits. For these reasons, the number of subjects necessarily varied from one analysis to the next.

The status of the coronary and control groups at the time of the follow-up was:

Coronary group (100 originally)	**Control group** (146 originally)
1 lost to follow-up	1 lost to follow-up
78 deceased	21 deceased (one of whom was re-examined, but died shortly thereafter)
21 living	124 living
20 examined	115 examined (10 were either uncooperative, out of the country, or disabled)

References

1 National Center for Health Statistics, Department of Health, Education, and Welfare, *Monthly Vital Statistics* Report, Provisional Statistics Annual Summary for the U.S., 1968, vol. 17, no. 13 (Washington, D.C.: U.S. Government Printing Office, 1969), p. 17.

2 National Health Education Committee Survey, *Facts on Major Killing and Crippling Diseases in U.S.,* (Rockville, Maryland: National Heart Institute, 1971), pp. 1-24.

3 M. M. Gertler, P. D. White et al., *Coronary Heart Disease in Young Adults.* The Commonwealth Fund (Cambridge: Harvard University Press, 1954).

II Development of Statistical Procedures in the Epidemiological Study of Coronary Heart Disease

Linear Regression Analysis

The 1951 communication, "Young Candidates for Coronary Heart Disease," by Gertler, Garn, and White, showed that a candidate for coronary heart disease (C.H.D.) could be selected from the putatively normal population.[1] This was accomplished by screening 100 coronary disease subjects and 146 randomly selected controls for factors that would distinguish between these two groups.

In addition to the marked differences found between the coronary and control groups with respect to chemistries and family histories, the anthropometric phase of the study revealed that the C.H.D. group exhibited a body build markedly different from that of the randomly selected controls. Because of this difference, it was thought that the best control group would be an individually matched group. Thus, an additional group of healthy men was selected on the basis of similar physical characteristics and ethnic backgrounds. When each of the variables was compared among the C.H.D. group, the randomly selected control group, and the matched control group, it was found that the greatest differences were between the C.H.D. group and the randomly selected control group (see Tables 2.1 and 2.2).[2]

Although the matched controls were significantly different from the coronaries, they also differed from the random controls. Both cholesterol esters and total cholesterol in the matched control group were significantly higher than in the randomly selected group. Therefore, the matched control group resembled the coronary group more closely than did the randomly selected controls.

It was reasoned that the matched control group would be more predisposed to C.H.D. than the random controls, since the matched controls were more similar to the C.H.D. group with respect to the characteristics separating the coronary group from the controls. This concept was presented to the New York Heart Association in 1949.

Following the presentation, it was thought that a more accurate method of selecting C.H.D. candidates from the normal population was necessary to identify those individuals who were incubating C.H.D. so that primary preventive programs could be instituted. In addition, it was important to obtain a group of coronary-prone individuals who could be studied further and more efficiently for additional risk factors that might prove to be more important than those already known.

Since it was found that C.H.D. was associated with multiple variables, rather than simply one, a technique was sought that would effectively correlate and weigh each parameter so that a more accurate classification could be made.

The statistical data up to that time were primarily based on a summation of

Table 2.1 Summary of the means and their standard errors of the four lipids and four indicial ratios of the control group, the coronary disease group, and the matched control group

	Control group	Coronary disease group	Matched control group
Free cholesterol	99.69 ± 2.33	110.36 ± 3.86	100.8 ± 3.90
Cholesterol esters	124.63 ± 2.6	176.66 ± 5.47	141.0 ± 3.88
Total cholesterol	224.42 ± 3.53	286.61 ± 6.50	241.9 ± 5.50
Phospholipids	200.32 ± 3.33	316.42 ± 6.7	305.7 ± 4.17
Cholesterol esters / Total cholesterol	55.61 ± 0.77	61.43 ± 1.06	58.5 ± 0.00
Free cholesterol / Total cholesterol	44.30 ± .76	38.57 ± 1.06	41.0 ± .97
Free cholesterol / Cholesterol esters	84.76 ± 2.47	68.10 ± 3.00	76.96 ± 2.99
Total cholesterol / Phospholipids	74.1 ± .92	80.4 ± 2.04	77.6 ± 1.32

Permission to reproduce granted by The American Heart Association, Inc. and M. M. Gertler, S. M. Garn, and J. Lerman, "The Interrelationships of Serum Cholesterol, Cholesterol Esters and Phospholipids in Health and in Coronary Artery Disease," *Circulation* II(2): 205-214, 1950.

Table 2.2 Serum uric acid in the control group, the coronary disease group, and the matched control group

Serum uric acid (mg. %)	Control group	Coronary disease group	Matched control group
2.5-2.9	1	0	0
3.0-3.4	4	5	2
3.5-3.9	20	9	8
4.0-4.4	38	15	24
4.5-4.9	38	19	23
5.0-5.4	23	14	20
5.5-5.9	13	10	13
6.0-6.4	7	6	4
6.5-6.9	2	6	2
7.0-7.4	0	5	0
7.5-7.9	0	3	0
Number	146	92	96
Mean ± standard error	4.64 ± .06	5.13 ± .12*	4.85 ± .07
Per cent above 5 mg per cent	31	48	42
Per cent above 6 mg per cent	6	22	6

*The differences of means between the coronary disease group and both of the other groups are highly significant (p=.01). The difference between the means of the control group and the matched control group is significant (p=.05).

Permission to reproduce granted by M. M. Gertler, S. M. Garn, and S. A. Levine, "Serum Uric Acid in Relation to Age and Physique in Health and in Coronary Heart Disease," *Ann. Int. Med.* 34: 1426, 1951.

individual abnormalities beyond a specific critical level. The essentials of this method were employed by several longitudinal studies (including cross-tabulation of two or three variables) until recently, when they yielded to the more modern and pertinent methodology to be described in this chapter.

The question of which particular combination of the variables studied would best discriminate between the two groups was subjected to precise quantitative evaluation with the use of a multiple linear regression analysis. This procedure was shown by Fisher to be equivalent to a discriminant function analysis when the dependent variable was chosen to be an appropriate dichotomous variable.[3] In this study, the variable to be predicted (the dependent variable) was chosen to be zero for the control group and 100 for the C.H.D. group. The predicting (independent) variables were biochemical, genetic, and other related factors that could be measured prior to the overt manifestations of the disease.

The discriminant function of the data derived by the above procedure included the following variables: height; weight; ponderal index (height over cube root of weight); total serum cholesterol level; ratio of total cholesterol and phospholipid levels; endomorphic index; mesomorphic index; ectomorphic index; and presence of coronary heart disease in mother, father, and sibling(s). This function was derived to calculate a score on each individual that would best distinguish between disease and control subjects.

The resulting discrimination was good, but it was believed that an improved analysis could be made by transforming the biochemical and physical measurements to logarithms, thus producing less variability in the data caused by the positively skewed distributions. Since the logarithmic function transformed a quotient into a difference of two terms, the various ratios could be replaced by the original individual variables. In the initial analysis there was a larger dispersion of discriminant scores within the coronary group than within the control group, reflecting the positive skew and the greater dispersion at the upper end of the distributions of the predicting variables. It was expected (and it proved to be the case) that this heterogeneity would be corrected in the second analysis by the use of logarithms (see *Results of analysis*). This was performed by the computing laboratory of the New York University College of Engineering, Research Division, under the direction of Dr. Max Woodbury.

The final equation was the function that best discriminated between the coronary and control groups. In the original data, using a dividing point of 37, and classifying subjects above 37 as coronary and below 37 as noncoronary, 81 per cent of the total group were correctly classified.[4]

The application of this equation in a new subject was made by measuring height, cholesterol, phospholipids, uric acid, mesomorphy, and family history. These measurements were entered into the equation, and the resulting score was calculated. A score close to zero indicated the subject was not coronary-prone. A score close to 100 indicated a high risk of coronary disease. Values between these two extremes were interpreted accordingly.

Examples of high-risk and low-risk subjects are given in Table 2.3 with the calculation of a profile score.

Results of a prospective study

The first test to determine the value of the linear regression equation in singling out

Results of analysis

Coronary discriminant analysis				Correlation coefficients	
X_1	Log of height			$X_{1.9}$	−0.29747
X_2	Log of total cholesterol level			$X_{2.9}$	+0.48992
X_3	Log of phospholipid level			$X_{3.9}$	+0.11189
X_4	Log of uric acid level			$X_{4.9}$	+0.24837
X_5	Mesomorphic index			$X_{5.9}$	+0.24796
	Disease in family			$X_{6.9}$	+0.21938
	Mother	Father	Siblings	$X_{7.9}$	+0.17081
X_6	+	+	—	$X_{8.9}$	+0.18548
X_7	+	–	+		
X_8	–	+	+		

$Y = X_9 = (100 = \text{coronary}, 0 = \text{control})$

Final equation in stepwise procedure

$$Y = 898.28 - 546.15X_1 + 218.29X_2 - 94.75X_3 + 63.19X_4 + 6.35X_5 + 38.86X_6 + 57.23X_7 + 48.4X_8$$

Order of selection of variables in regression

$X_2, X_6, X_1, X_7, X_5, X_3, X_8, X_4$

Permission to reproduce granted by The American Heart Association, Inc. and M. M. Gertler, M. A. Woodbury, L. G. Gottsch et al., "The Candidate For Coronary Heart Disease," *JAMA* 170: 151, 1959.

Table 2.3 Calculations of profile score

	High-risk subject	Low-risk subject
Height (inches)	66	73
Cholesterol (mg. %)	295	210
Phospholipids (mg. %)	11.2	9.1
Uric acid (mg. %)	6.1	4.9
Mesomorphy	6	4
Family history		
Mother	+	–
Father	+	–
Siblings	+	–
Profile score*	116.7	11.5

*Profile score calculated by the final equation in *Results of analysis.*

the candidate for ischemic heart disease took place in 1959 in New York City in an industrial population.[5] The prospective study included 490 men between the ages of 23 and 79. They were in good health and free from any overt disease at the time of the examination. The profile score for each individual was determined at the outset of the study and the group was periodically followed over the course of 10 years. The group considered to be highly prone to C.H.D. was selected on the basis of a score above the mean + 1.3 standard deviation (62.2) of the profile score. This value was chosen because it was exceeded by 50 per cent of the coronary cases and less than 3 per cent of the controls in the original 1949 study. Using this critical level, 32 men were chosen as candidates for C.H.D. from the total of 490 men. The other 458 members were not considered high-risk at the time of the first examination. A follow-up study in 1964 revealed that 28 out of these 32 cases came down with either angina pectoris and/or acute C.H.D., while not one of the 458 experienced C.H.D. or angina pectoris. The follow-up in 1972 revealed that all 32 of the disease-prone group experienced C.H.D. while only 12 members of the nonprone group of 458 had experienced C.H.D. Seven of these 12 men experienced elevated serum cholesterol and uric acid levels, which increased the value of their profile scores. The remaining five men died before data were obtained, so it would be difficult to assess their status with regard to profile score.

Statistical procedures

Early studies of C.H.D. were directed toward the recognition of factors associated with the disease and an understanding of the defects responsible for its development.

In general, there are two major types of epidemiological studies that have been designed and reported. The first type, to which this study belongs, is retrospective. For studies of this nature, a group of coronary heart disease subjects are selected and compared with a group of controls selected in a manner similar to the disease subjects.

Other studies have been prospective by design. For these, a study population is chosen within the age range of individuals considered susceptible to coronary heart disease. The variables thought to be associated with the disease are then measured at regular intervals for each individual. In the study group, analysis is made on the data after a sufficient number in the cohort have developed the disease. This provides the investigator with a group of disease subjects and controls with data measurements before the onset of the disease. Factors associated with the disease are selected primarily by categorizing the data according to the variables measured, then comparing the morbidity rate of the disease at various levels of these measurements.

Data from retrospective studies have been analyzed primarily by means of comparison of the prevalence of abnormalities between the diseased and control groups. Dichotomous variables (those with only two possible outcomes, such as family history, history of associated diseases, or other discrete abnormalities) yield well to this analysis. However, many studies have utilized this technique for continuous variables by selecting an arbitrary critical level above which that variable is considered abnormal. The insensitivity of this procedure may best be seen by an example: If 260 mg per cent were considered the critical level for serum cholesterol, a subject with a cholesterol level of 255 mg per cent would be considered normal, whereas another subject with a level of 265 mg per cent would be abnormal, indicating an increased level of risk. Continuous variables can be compared by use of the student's t-test for significant differences, and, more recently, logistic functions of continuous variables have been applied to explore the actual relationship between the variables and risk of C.H.D.

Another weakness in some early reports of epidemiological studies is their failure to assess the interrelationships between the various risk factors. Multiple cross-classification has been used primarily for this analysis, but the weakness of this procedure has been described: "If 10 variables are under consideration, and each variable is to be studied at only three levels . . . there would be 59,049 cells in the multiple cross-classification."[6] It is evident that extensive multivariate analysis by cross-classification becomes prohibitive for even a small number of variables. However, Keys (1971) refutes the futility of this situation by suggesting a careful choice of variables to be included in a cross-classification. If one includes only those variables with theoretical or empirical importance and excludes those variables that are highly correlated with one another, that is, diastolic and systolic blood pressure (which would minimize redundant effects), the number of cells and, thus, subjects can be made manageable.[7]

The possibility of combining the individual risk factors into a joint measure of risk was first reported by this group in 1959. This attempt was prompted by the desire to find a function of those factors associated with coronary heart disease that would discriminate between the coronary and control groups better than any single individual factor. The procedure used was the multivariate discriminant function analysis previously described.

In 1962, Cornfield published an analysis of the joint dependence of risk of coronary heart disease in Framingham on two variables: serum cholesterol and systolic blood pressure.[8] In addition, he utilized the model of discriminant functions to find a linear function of these two variables. Using an application of Bayes' formula, a transformation of the discriminant function into the multiple logistic equation was made that yielded a probability of developing the disease rather than merely discriminating between the two groups. By comparing the calculated probability of C.H.D. from the 95th percentile to the 5th percentile, that is, the top 5 per cent to the bottom 5 per cent for either cholesterol or systolic blood pressure individually, an almost fivefold increase in risk was found. The joint risk ratio for an individual with both cholesterol and systolic blood pressure at the 95th percentile as compared to the 5th percentile was almost 25-fold. This demonstrates the value of jointly assessing the risk factors associated with coronary heart disease.

An extension of the procedure described by Cornfield was reported in 1967 by Truett et al.[9] A discriminant function of seven variables was calculated based on the 12-year experience of the Framingham Study. The risk factors included were age, cholesterol, systolic blood pressure, relative weight, hemoglobin, cigarette smoking, and ECG abnormalities. Once again, the discriminant function was utilized in the multiple logistic equation in order to give a probability of C.H.D., that is, $P=1/[1+\exp(-\alpha-\Sigma\beta_i X_i)]$. One important question that was answered by this publication was whether data not meeting the multivariate normal assumptions could be fitted by a discriminant function based on this assumption—that is, whether each of the variables was normally distributed. It was found that as long as the discriminant function of the independent variables was univariate normal, this was a sufficient condition to fit the data with a discriminant function. This agreement was demonstrated by comparing the observed number of C.H.D. cases in each decile of risk to the expected number, where the expected number was found by summing the calculated probabilities for each subject within the decile.

Other than age, the risk factors found to be most important were cholesterol, cigarette smoking, ECG abnormalities, and systolic blood pressure. In comparing the risk rate between the highest and lowest deciles of risk from all factors, a 30-fold increase was found for men and 70-fold increase for women. These relative differences were largest at younger ages in both men and women.

In 1967, another publication by Walker and Duncan described a method of estimating the coefficients for the multiple logistic equation for dichotomous or polychotomous data.[10] No assumptions about the underlying distributions were made, and the coefficients were calculated by a recursive technique. This procedure can be utilized when the dependent variable has two possible outcomes: myocardial infarction or angina pectoris, or no C.H.D., for example. In both instances, the function calculates a probability of a particular outcome from the independent predictors or risk factors.

The multivariate procedures described here have been the most powerful tools for combining the joint effect of the various risk factors characteristic of C.H.D. A single estimate of disease proneness can be made for any individual by accounting for both the direct relationship of the characteristic to the disease and the interrelationship between the various characteristics. Thus, the population sector at highest risk of C.H.D. can be identified.

Other Risk Factor Studies

From 1948 and extending into the 1970s, a number of long-term prospective coronary heart disease studies were initiated to verify that characteristics associated with C.H.D. actually occurred prior to the onset of the overt manifestation of the disease. Each of these studies was designed and pursued by independent investigators, and, therefore, various aspects of these studies are not comparable. Among the various studies, different laboratory assay methods were used, and several different diagnostic criteria of coronary heart disease were employed. As a result of their independence, however, common results or findings from several studies lend special credibility. In this brief section, these results will be summarized.

The studies we will review here are the Framingham Study,[11] the Los Angeles Study,[12] the Chicago Study,[13] and the Albany Study,[14]—all of which followed over 1,500 subjects and began before 1960. Also included are the Chicago Utility Company Study,[15] the Western Collaborative Group Study,[16] and the Minnesota Study.[17]

The Framingham Study

The Framingham Study began in 1948 to investigate arteriosclerotic and hypertensive cardiovascular disease, primarily to isolate and define the constitutional and conditioning factors that precede their occurrence. A cohort of approximately 4,500 subjects, aged 30-59 years, was selected for the study and followed for 20 years.

The variables measured on each biennial examination were: systolic blood pressure, diastolic blood pressure, cholesterol, hemoglobin, phospholipids, blood sugar, uric acid, relative weight, vital capacity, alcohol and cigarette consumption, urine albumin and sugar, heart enlargement, ECG, presence of diabetes mellitus, hypertension, and glucose intolerance.

The five characteristics from the above measurements that make a joint contribution to a multiple risk function are systolic blood pressure, cholesterol, cigarette smoking, glucose intolerance, and ECG abnormality left ventricular hypertrophy (L.V.H.). The multivariate analysis of the relationship of cardiovascular disorders to the various characteristics or risk factors measured is described in Section 27 of the Framingham Study. The procedure utilized was that proposed by Walker and Duncan (1967), which computes the coefficients of the logistic risk equation.

The five key variables mentioned above were found most important in discriminating between those who would and those who would not develop the three most important atherothrombotic events considered: coronary heart disease, atherothrombotic brain infarction, and intermittent claudication. For each of these events and for the different age groups, a risk function was calculated that best described the data.

The Los Angeles Study

The Los Angeles Study (Chapman et al., 1957) of coronary heart disease was initiated in 1949. The sample selected from city civil service employes consisted of 2,252 persons in the age range of 18-70 years. The subjects were examined at intervals of 12 to 18 months. Each subject completed a history questionnaire and was given a physical examination, X-ray, ECG, and fluoroscopy of the chest. Also, vital capacity, urine analysis, blood count, sedimentation rate, hematocrit, blood sugar, and serum cholesterol were measured on each subject.

The prevalence of coronary heart disease was found to be 2.7 per cent of the male sample. The incidence of new heart disease in the study was assessed by observing the 1,653 males who were diagnosed as having normal hearts on entry into the study. For males aged 40-54 years, the incidence was 8 per 1,000; for males 55-70 years, the incidence was 29 per 1,000.

Systolic blood pressure above 145 and diastolic above 95 mm Hg was associated with increased incidence of C.H.D. in the age range 40-54 years. In the older age group, however, no association with blood pressure was evidenced. The statistical analysis of data in this report was accomplished by simply tabulating the number of cases and calculating percentages for various levels of each variable. Except for age stratification, no attempt was made to investigate interrelationships between variables.

The Chicago Study

A cohort of males aged 40-55, employed at the Hawthorne Works of the Western Electric Company, was selected for a longitudinal study of coronary heart disease (Paul et al., 1963). After the first year of examinations there were 1,989 participants.

Information recorded for each study subject consisted of a complete personal and family history, diet estimates, physical activity, X-ray, ECG, urinalysis, hemoglobin, cholesterol, skinfolds, somatotype, lipoprotein, B.P., and psychological measures.

Incidence of coronary heart disease was 10/1,000 annually over the 4½ years followed at this report. No association was found between the age at which parents died and coronary disease in the subjects. Subjects with histories of either chest discomfort, cough, shortness of breath, or peptic ulcer had a higher incidence of C.H.D. than those without these characteristics.

Skinfold measurements were significantly larger in the coronary group, indicating relative fatness in this group, although height and weight showed no differences. The somatotype measures revealed that the coronary group was predominantly endomorphic.

Systolic blood pressure, and to a lesser extent diastolic blood pressure, was related to the incidence of C.H.D. The mean cholesterol level was significantly higher in the coronary group than in the noncoronary group.

The data on smoking habits showed a strong relationship between the number of cigarettes smoked and C.H.D. This relationship held for both current smoking habits and smoking habits for most of a subject's adult life.

Although the authors recognize that C.H.D. is a multifactorial disease, the statistical analysis employed in this report considered only individual variables and their association with C.H.D.

The Albany Study

The New York State Department of Health, in conjunction with the Albany Medical College, began a Cardiovascular Health Center in 1953 for the study of degenerative cardiovascular disease (Doyle et al., 1959). Volunteer male civil service employes, aged 39-55 years, entered into the study. The initial examination included a complete medical and family history, a physical examination, urinalysis, X-ray, ECG, and stress test ECG. Skinfold measurements were made, and laboratory studies included hemoglobin and serum total cholesterol. At this report, 653 subjects had been followed for 44 months. The prevalence of ischemic heart disease found at the start of the study was 37 per 1,000.

The average annual incidence of ischemic heart disease, myocardial infarction, and angina pectoris was 8.5 per 1,000 in the male group aged 40-54 years.

No association was found between family history of vascular disease and ischemic heart disease in the subjects. In addition, no association was found between somatotype classification and ischemic heart disease incidence among smokers versus nonsmokers.

The only association found between ischemic heart disease and blood pressure was when diastolic blood pressure had risen above 110 mm Hg. A twofold increased incidence of ischemic heart disease was found with subjects 40 per cent or more overweight. A threefold increase in incidence was found when cholesterol was over 275 mg per cent.

The above-mentioned analyses were made individually. However, the report states that the combination of two or three abnormalities of diastolic blood pressure, serum total cholesterol, and relative body weight did not significantly compound the risk with any of these individual abnormalities.

The Chicago Utility Company Study

In 1954, an epidemiological program (Stamler et al., 1960) was begun in a Chicago utility corporation, the People's Gas Company, to study the occurrence, natural history, and etiology of hypertensive and atherosclerotic cardiovascular diseases. Complete medical records were available on 756 men aged 50-59 years as of Jan. 1, 1954. Follow-up examinations on most subjects were available for the 4 years through Dec. 31, 1957, and, except for 16 subjects, the status of the cohort's health was known at the close of the follow-up period.

The routine examinations consisted of a medical history, physical examination, urinalysis, ECG, and chest X-ray. Available data from these examinations included weight, height, blood pressure, and sociologic information. The incidence of new coronary heart disease during the 4 years among the males aged 50-59 was 61/1,000 or 15/1,000 annually. Analysis of the various factors associated with coronary heart disease was accomplished by stratification of these factors and comparison of the incidence rates within the subcategories.

Subjects with relative weight over 113, that is, 13 per cent above median weight for height, were designated as markedly obese and found to be associated with a doubling of incidence of C.H.D. when compared with subjects below the relative weight of 100.

Subjects with hypertension were found to have an almost threefold higher incidence than normotensive subjects. The joint effect of obesity and hypertension was measured by cross-tabulating these two factors. The incidence of C.H.D. in subjects with both characteristics was almost four times what it was for those with neither.

Stratification of the data by sociologic variables yielded a lower C.H.D. incidence rate among semiskilled and unskilled workers, although not significantly lower.

Both prevalence and incidence rates of C.H.D. were twice as great for diabetics as for nondiabetics.

This study was based on information derived from existing medical records of an industrial population. By careful evaluation of these records, the disease incidence and prevalence could be accurately assessed, and physical characteristics determined. The shortcomings of this method lay in the omissions from the medical record of variables known to be important in the development of the disease. These included cholesterol levels and smoking history, among others.

The Western Collaborative Group Study

The Western Collaborative Group Study (Rosenman et al., 1970) was initiated in 1960, much later than the other large prospective studies, and followed 3,182 men from 4 to 5 years.

One important aspect of this study was the typing of behavior patterns into Type A, characterized by an excessive sense of time urgency, aggressiveness, and competitive drive; and Type B, those who didn't have these characteristics.

Analysis of the study was made by comparing the coronary and noncoronary groups in terms of the characteristics measured at the initiation of the study. These comparisons were made for each variable individually. In addition, the joint effects of two variables at a time were analyzed to assess the interaction between the independent variables.

The analysis made of these data was well suited to the dichotomous variables (for example, smoking, history of disease, behavioral type, etc.) since comparisons between the groups were made with chi square analysis. However, continuous variables such as blood pressure and cholesterol were dichotomized into two ranges using appropriate clinical criteria to determine the cutoff between normal and abnormal levels. As described earlier, this procedure is not the most powerful method of analysis since it is insensitive to broad changes in each category, whereas a small change across the critical point causes a total reclassification of the subject. The variables found to be significantly associated with C.H.D. when analyzed singly were educational level, family history of C.H.D., history of hypertension, history of diabetes mellitus, cigarettes smoked per day, systolic and diastolic blood pressure, cholesterol, triglycerides, lipoprotein classification, and behavior type. However, when the above variables were analyzed jointly on the risk of coronary heart disease (that is, the joint effect of two variables at a time on the incidence of disease) the cholesterol and lipoprotein measures were dependent on each other, as were the cholesterol and triglyceride measures. The effect of cholesterol, however, was independent of that of diastolic blood pressure; family history was independent of behavioral type; and cholesterol was independent of behavioral type. In an attempt to verify the fact that behavioral type was a significant factor in C.H.D. incidence, the effects of 12 other variables were held statistically constant by the use of a multiple regression. By utilizing this procedure, the association between behavior type and C.H.D. was found to exist independently of the other 12 risk factors.

The Minnesota Study

This study of coronary heart disease was made on 279 middle-aged business and professional men, aged 45-55 at the start of the study (Keys et al., 1971). The study began in 1947, but at this report, using the three initial annual examinations to establish baseline levels for the study characteristics, the follow-up is the 20-year period from 1950 through 1970.

The annual examination consisted of the following: blood pressure, height, weight, ECG, urinalysis, skinfolds, total serum cholesterol, hemoglobin, vital capacity, protein-bound iodine, a medical and family history, and a cardiovascular questionnaire. During the third year of follow-up, the cold pressor test was administered to each subject.

Analysis of the 20-year follow-up was made both with single-variable and multi-variate analysis. Each of the single variables was either dichotomized or trichotomized and the incidence of new disease compared among several levels of each characteristic. The individual variables found to be significantly associated with C.H.D. were smoking habit, systolic blood pressure, cholesterol, and the cold pressor test.

To investigate the multivariate relationship of the primary risk factors to C.H.D., Walker and Duncan's method (1967) was used to calculate the coefficients of the multiple logistic function. The effectiveness of this function in describing the data was tested by calculating the probability within each decile of risk. The sum of the probabilities then reflected the expected number of cases for that decile. The observed number of cases was plotted against the expected number within each decile, and the correlation coefficient of these points reflected the ability of the model to describe the data. This procedure was followed for five variables, that is, cholesterol, systolic blood pressure, cold pressor rise, smoking habit, and body mass index (weight/height squared). Several additional functions were calculated using subsets of these variables to investigate the independence and necessity of these variables (for example, using systolic blood pressure, cholesterol, and cold pressor rise, but omitting body mass index and smoking habit).

A correlation of .86 was found between observed and expected numbers of C.H.D. death and myocardial infarction using all five of the above variables. For all C.H.D. incidents, including angina pectoris, a correlation of .78 was obtained. Averaging the observed number of incidents of death or myocardial infarction within the lowest and highest quintile of estimated risk by four different risk functions yielded 1.5 cases in the lowest and 16.75 cases in the highest, or a ratio of 1 to 11. Therefore, by selecting subjects in the highest 20 per cent of estimated risk and the lowest 20 per cent, an 11-fold difference in the number of C.H.D. incidents would be expected.

This study of C.H.D., although small compared to several others, yielded results in basic agreement with others concerning cholesterol and blood pressure. The results of the smoking habit data, however, revealed that men smoking occasionally or regularly less

Table 2.4 Summary of variables studied by various investigators

Variable	Framingham	Los Angeles (Chapman)	Albany (Doyle)	Chicago (Paul)	Chicago (Stamler)	Western Collaborative	Minnesota (Keys)
Cholesterol	X*	X	X*	X*		X*	X*
Lipid phosphorus	X						
Triglycerides						X*	
Lipoproteins			X	X		X*	
Uric acid	X						
Hemoglobin	X		X	X			X
Fasting blood sugar							
Two-hour sugar				X			
Casual blood sugar	X*	X*					
Blood pressure	X*	X*	X*	X*	X	X*	X*
Height	X	X		X	X*	X	X
Weight	X	X		X	X	X*	X
Relative weight	X*		X*		X*		X
Ponderal index		X				X	
Somatotype				X			X
Vital capacity	X	X					
Alcohol	X						
Cigarettes	X*			X*		X*	X*
Urine albumin	X	X	X	X	X		
Urine sugar	X	X	X	X	X		
ECG	X	X	X	X*	X		X
Diabetes	X				X*	X*	
Hypertension	X				X	X*	
Family history		X	X	X*		X*	X
X-ray	X	X	X	X	X		X
Sedimentation rate		X					
Physical exam		X	X	X	X		
Hematocrit		X					
Diet				X			
Exercise		X		X		X	
Skinfolds			X	X*			X
Psychological				X		X*	
Coffee				X*			
Socio-economic					X	X	
P.B.I.							X
Cold pressor							X*
Chest discomfort				X*			
Chronic cough				X*			
Shortness of breath				X*			
Peptic ulcer				X*			
Blood count		X					
Stress test			X				
Education						X*	
Income						X	

*Indicates factors associated with incidence of C.H.D. according to the specific study.

than 10 cigarettes per day had the lowest incidence rate of coronary heart disease of all groups, including those who never smoked and those who had stopped smoking. Relative body weight in this study was shown to be unimportant in risk of C.H.D.

The logistic equation computed from these data was employed to estimate the risk for another independent sample. The predicted risk was then compared with the actual observed risk.

Though not perfect, the agreement between the observed and expected number of C.H.D. subjects in the sample was impressive.

Table 2.4 gives a summary of the different variables studied by investigators and elucidates one of the reasons for the ofttimes inconsistent findings reported.

Summary

The use of statistical analysis in public health surveys is not new. Attempts by actuarial departments in large insurance companies to determine survival rates for the population with coronary disease were the first statistical analyses to be attempted in this area. However, the statistical appraisal of coronary heart disease during the incubation period was not possible until the risk factors were ascertained and the degree of importance of each risk factor was studied by itself and in association with the others. This was not feasible until their publication in 1959 in the Journal of the American Medical Association, based on the data derived from the original study group reported in this monograph. This type of analysis describes the relationship of the risk factors to each other and, in addition, describes the contribution of each factor in numerical terms. The order of importance of the risk factors found in this statistical analysis was cholesterol, family history of heart disease, height, mesomorphy, phospholipids, and uric acid.

The 1959 publication stimulated further epidemiological studies, and many authors confirmed the original premises, albeit by modifying the methodology or increasing the number of observations. Some studies found cigarette smoking to play a major role in the etiology of coronary heart disease, while our analysis revealed that cigarettes played a minor role. Hypertension, for example, was considered by some investigators to be a strong factor, while others considered it to be of little significance, a finding that we share. Another factor over which there is disagreement is diabetes mellitus, which some believe to be a strong factor. We found, however, that its strength as a factor was more closely linked with stroke than coronary heart disease.

In a further statistical development, the multiple discriminant function was transformed to a multiple logistic function that made possible a probabilistic view of coronary risk based on a population sample. This probabilistic view was tested by many long-term epidemiological studies revealing comparable incidence rates. The Los Angeles Study reported an annual incidence of 8/1,000 in males aged 40-54 years. The Albany Study reported practically identical findings of 8.5/1,000 for men in the same age category. Similarly, Paul's Chicago Study showed a 10/1,000 incidence rate for males aged 40-55. Two study groups reporting on older populations revealed a 15/1,000 and 29/1,000 incidence rate for 50-59-year-old and 55-70-year-old males, respectively.

Further analysis of these large risk factor studies revealed many differences in the approach to the study of coronary heart disease. Among these differences were laboratory assay methods, diagnostic criteria for coronary heart disease, and statistical procedures. The variables most frequently analyzed in relation to heart disease were cholesterol, blood pressure, height, weight, ECG abnormalities, and chest X-rays. Table 2.4 points out the major differences in the study of risk factors.

The concept of identifying the candidate for coronary heart disease is now fully accepted. The concept of assessing the degree of risk is also becoming firmly established, as judged by the pamphlets on risk assessment based on actual arithmetical evaluations issued by the National Institutes of Health and the American Heart Association.

Recently, we extended our original concept to the selection of the candidate for ischemic thrombotic cerebrovascular disease (ITCVD), and found that the risk factors for ITCVD differ in both degree and substance from that of C.H.D., that is, diabetes mellitus is a major risk factor in ITCVD but not in C.H.D.

References

1 M. M. Gertler, S. M. Garn, and P. D. White, "Young Candidates for Coronary Heart Disease," *JAMA* 147: 621-625, 1951.

2 M. M. Gertler, S. M. Garn, and J. Lerman, "The Interrelationships of Serum Cholesterol, Cholesterol Esters and Phospholipids in Health and in Coronary Artery Disease," *Circulation* II(2): 205-214, 1950; M. M. Gertler, S. M. Garn, and S. A. Levine, "Serum Uric Acid in Relation to Age and Physique in Health and in Coronary Heart Disease," *Ann. Int. Med.* 34: 1421-1431, 1951.

3 R. A. Fisher, *Statistical Methods for Research Workers* (New York: Hafner, 1954), p. 285.

4 M. M. Gertler, M. A. Woodbury, L. G. Gottsch, P. D. White, and H. A. Rusk, "The Candidate for Coronary Heart Disease," *JAMA* 170: 149-152, 1959.

5 M. M. Gertler, P. D. White, L. D. Cady, and H. H. Whiter, "Coronary Heart Disease: A Prospective Study," *Am. J. Med. Sci.* 248: 377-398, 1964.

6 J. Truett, J. Cornfield, and W. B. Kannel, "A Multivariate Analysis of the Risk of Coronary Heart Disease in Framingham," *J. Chron. Dis.* 20: 511-524, 1964.

7 A. Keys, H. L. Taylor, H. Blackburn, J. Brozek, J. T. Anderson, and E. Simonson, "Mortality and Coronary Heart Disease Among Men Studied for 23 Years," *Arch. Int. Med.* 128: 201-214, 1971.

8 J. Cornfield, "Joint Dependence of Risk of Coronary Heart Disease on Serum Cholesterol and Systolic Blood Pressure: A Discriminant Function Analysis," *Fed. Proc.* 21: 58-61, 1962.

9 Truett et al., "A Multivariate Analysis," pp. 511-524.

10 S. H. Walker and D. B. Duncan, "Estimation of the Probability of an Event as a Function of Several Independent Variables," *Biometrika* 54: 167-179, 1967.

11 W. B. Kannel and T. Gordon, eds., *The Framingham Study: An Epidemiologic Investigation of Cardiovascular Diseases,* Section 26, Dec. 1970; Section 27, May 1971 (Washington, D.C.: U.S. Government Printing Office).

12 J. M. Chapman, C. S. Goerke, W. Dixon, D. B. Loveland, and E. Phillips, "The Clinical Status of a Population Group in Los Angeles Under Observation for Two to Three Years," *Am. J. Pub. Health* 47 (4): 33-42, 1957.

13 J. Stamler, H. A. Lindberg, D. M. Berkson et al., "Prevalence and Incidence of Coronary Heart Disease in Strata of Labor Force of a Chicago Industrial Population," *J. Chron. Dis.* II: 405-420, 1960.

14 J. T. Doyle, A. S. Heslin, H. E. Hilleboe, and P. F. Formel, "Early Diagnosis of Ischemic Heart Disease," *New Eng. J. Med.* 261: 1096-1101, 1959.

15 O. Paul, M. H. Lepper, W. H. Phelan et al., "A Longitudinal Study of Coronary Heart Disease," *Circulation* 28: 20-31, 1963.

16 R. H. Rosenman, M. Friedman, R. Strauss et al., "Coronary Heart Disease in the Western Collaborative Group Study," *J. Chron. Dis.* 23: 173-190, 1970.

17 Keys et al., "Mortality and Coronary Heart Disease," pp. 201-214.

III Clinical Appraisal of the Coronary Group

The purpose of this chapter is to describe the original 100 coronary heart disease patients studied with respect to such variables as sex, age, and occupation; to analyze the character and mode of onset of both the premonitory and acute prodromal symptoms; and to compare the initial 1949 clinical findings on both subjects and controls with the findings of 1971. Wherever possible, reasons for differences, as well as their significance, are discussed.

Composition of the Group

Sex

Of the 100 patients examined in 1949, 97 were men and three were women. In 1971, there were 20 males and one female remaining out of the original coronary group, virtually the same proportion as was observed in 1949.

Age

The three women examined in 1949 were 35, 39, and 40 years of age. The ages of the 97 men at the time of the acute episodes ranged from 22-40 years, the average being 35.4 years. There were eight men 22-29 years old, inclusive; 28 men 30-34 years old, inclusive; and 61 men 35-40 years old, inclusive. The age at the time of examination ranged from 24-51 years, with an average of 38.2 years. The lapse of time between onset of myocardial infarction and our examination is given in Table 3.1.

Of the original 100 coronary patients, there were 21 remaining subjects as of 1971–20 male survivors and one female. Five of the male survivors were between the ages of 48 and 52 years, seven were between 57 and 60, and eight were between 61 and 68. The one female survivor was 60 years of age. The average age of the male survivors was 59, which indicates an average survival period of approximately 24 years since the first coronary episode. Unfortunately, one surviving coronary subject was not available for a follow-up examination.

Race

The question as to whether one can be "racially predisposed" to coronary heart disease is far from answered. The selection of patients for study, the origin of the various reports, and the interpretation of the final results all complicate the issue.

Nearly all the ethnic groups on the East Coast (the home of 70 per cent of the patients) were represented in this series. The progenitors, both male and female, of nearly half the group originated in the British Isles. Individuals of Mediterranean or Eastern Mediterranean origin comprised 37 per cent of the entire group, a proportion well in

Table 3.1 Lapse of time between onset of myocardial infarction and initial examination of 97 male patients

Years	Number of patients	Years	Number of patients
0.5-1.0	17	5.51-6.0	3
1.01-1.5	14	6.01-6.5	3
1.51-2.0	15	6.51-7.0	3
2.01-2.5	8	7.01-7.5	4
2.51-3.0	8	7.51-8.0	2
3.01-3.5	2	8.01-9.0	3
3.51-4.0	4	9.01-10.0	2
4.01-4.5	3	10.01-11.0	0
4.51-5.0	4	11.01-12.0	1
5.01-5.5	0	26.01-27.0*	1

*This man was examined by the late Dr. H. B. Sprague in 1923.

Permission to reproduce granted by Harvard University Press and M. M. Gertler, P. D. White, *Coronary Heart Disease in Young Adults* (Cambridge: Harvard University Press, 1954), p. 9. Copyright 1954 by The Commonwealth Fund.

excess of their percentage representation in the areas from which the sample was drawn.[1]

Occupation

Several reports in the literature have been concerned with a causal relationship between coronary heart disease and occupational pursuits.[2] It has been found that an excessive number of patients with C.H.D. fall into certain occupational categories. Upon analyzing the occupational breakdown of the original male coronary group of 97, it was found that the managerial category embraced 43 per cent, the semiprofessional category 7 per cent, the professional category (including doctors) 11 per cent, the semiskilled category 31 per cent, the skilled labor category 4 per cent, and the unskilled labor category 3 per cent. Thus, in this limited series as in other more extensive series, certain types of occupations were found to predominate. But it is important to note that at the original examination a large proportion were already private and not clinic patients. Of the 20 surviving male coronary patients, seven were in managerial positions, while in 1949 only two were managers.

This increase may be due to many things, one of which is the element of seniority. Coronary heart disease, it should be noted, does not mitigate against the acceptance and execution of greater responsibility. Table 3.2 shows the death rate of the total coronary group in the various occupational categories.

It is sobering to observe that over 95 per cent of the men in the managerial category were not surviving in 1971. The managerial and semiskilled groups had the highest death rates in our study. There is something contradictory in these observations, however. The semiskilled individual is usually physically active and should, on the basis of activity, show less recurrence. On the other hand, managerial positions are usually filled by intense and persistent individuals who desire recognition and advancement, and who work under the pressure of time limits, making them excellent candidates for C.H.D.

The death rates in the professional, semiprofessional, and skilled categories are 50-57 per cent. However, the original numbers are too small to draw any conclusion.

Table 3.2 Death rates in relation to various occupational levels in original male coronary group

Occupational category	Per cent 1949	Number deceased	Per cent deceased
Managerial	43	40	95
Semiprofessional	7	4	57
Professional	11	6	55
Semiskilled	31	24	80
Skilled	4	2	50
Unskilled	3	0	0

Incidence and Symptoms

Incidence of infarction

When the incidence of infarction was studied in terms of the time of occurrence, it was found that the majority of acute coronary events took place during the hours of increased activity, with the greatest incidence in the early afternoon. There was a decline in the rate of occurrence of myocardial infarction between 6 P.M. and 6 A.M., when only 34 per cent of the coronary group experienced their attacks, while 66 per cent of the group experienced their myocardial infarctions between 6 A.M. and 6 P.M. The data concerning the relationship between recurrent episodes and the time of day were not significantly different from the original findings.

Symptoms

Of the 64 patients who gave a history of symptoms that preceded the acute episode, eight said the complaints had been present for more than a year. Of these eight, three gave indigestion as a symptom, two nervousness, and three angina pectoris. Three others complained of having had indigestion and nervousness for as long as four years; one reported dyspnea for as long as five years. The 52 remaining patients noted having had some form of distress (angina pectoris in 38 cases) for less than a year, in most cases for only a few months. Three of the 38 who had had angina pectoris for less than a year suffered tightness in the chest on exertion for only three days before the acute attack, symptoms which may represent a partial occlusion of one of the coronary vessels progressing, with continued activity, to complete occlusion and infarction.

It is noteworthy that only four of the original 100 patients suffered no pain during the acute episode, although they did have other complaints. The other 96 patients did experience chest pains. Among the other major complaints were nausea, indigestion, dyspnea, vomiting, and excessive sweating. Five or fewer patients experienced dizziness, weakness, cyanosis, headache, palpitations, and choking. The pain, when experienced, lasted an average of six hours, with extreme variations of from 20 minutes to 72 hours.

The locations to which the chest pain radiated were not always the classical sites; in less than half of the instances of radiated chest pain (29 out of 68 patients) did the pain radiate down both arms. In 28 cases there was chest pain with no radiation.

There was no significant change in the type or duration of symptomatology in subsequent episodes experienced by the coronary group from those reported for the first acute episode.

Table 3.3 Distribution by month of acute episodes of myocardial infarction in coronary patients

Month	Number of episodes Original study	Follow-up study
January	13	3
February	4	4
March	11	3
April	5	3
May	13	8
June	1	1
July	7	2
August	4	6
September	10	9
October	9	4
November	12	6
December	11	2

Activity at onset of acute episode

Of the 18 patients listed as having had their major attacks while performing manual labor, nine were engaged in some type of work to which they were not accustomed. In two of these cases, unusual excitement on top of the unusual activity may have been a contributory factor. A total of 21 patients were engaged in some type of activity—exercise or otherwise—that required greater work on the part of the heart than was required by their usual daily routine. This may have been a factor in the development of infarction of the myocardium, at least in some patients. Of the 100 cases, one-third were resting or sleeping at the onset of acute myocardial infarction.

Again, the analysis of the activity patterns revealed no significant differences between the initial episode and subsequent episodes.

Distribution of episodes by season and month

The distribution of the episodes into the months and/or seasons did not support the contention that there is a seasonal proclivity to the coronary episodes. The summary of the subsequent episodes is listed in Table 3.3 and compared with the original episodes. A similar conclusion can be drawn from analysis of the monthly episodes of the controls.

The combined colder weather months (those comprising fall and winter) accounted for 60 per cent of the cases originally studied and only 43 per cent of the episodes in the follow-up study. There was no significant seasonal preponderance with respect to incidence of episodes of C.H.D. in the control group, except that nine of the 16 events fell between the months of June and August.

Subsequent episodes in the coronary group

Table 3.4 summarizes the total number of episodes experienced by the coronary group and the average number of years survived by those who experienced various numbers of attacks.

Fifty-two per cent of the C.H.D. group had at least one additional attack. Thirty-four per cent experienced two episodes, while 8 per cent experienced a third. Six per cent experienced four attacks, and 3 per cent had five attacks. Of the entire group who expe-

*Table 3.4 Summary of original and subsequent coronary episodes within coronary group of 99**

Number of episodes	Number of cases	Deceased	Alive	Mean survival (years)
1	48	32	16	9.4
2	34	32	2	11.4
3	8	6	2	11.6
4	6	6	0	13.5
5	3	2	1	18.5

*One coronary subject was lost to follow-up.

rienced one episode, 16 are still living; two of the 34 subjects who experienced two attacks are still living; and one subject who experienced five episodes is still alive. In the control group, 23 individuals developed C.H.D. There have been no subsequent attacks within the control group.

Mortality in the coronary group

It was thought that a long-term follow-up would yield more definite survival and mortality information than speculation alone could provide, as well as offer the chance to correlate the length of survival with various parameters to determine whether specific therapeutic intervention would be helpful.

The causes of death in the coronary group are listed in Table 3.5. The post-coronary survival pattern of the 78 deceased subjects is given in Table 3.6 based on five-year intervals. The graph in Figure 3.1 exemplifies this pattern in a continuous moving survival curve.

The mortality picture of our group of coronary subjects cannot really be compared to other series because this group was selected according to age (that is, under 40 at the time of the coronary attack) and lack of specific diseases (that is, hypertension, overt diabetes mellitus, xanthomatosis, hypo- and hyperthyroidism). These cases were in

Table 3.5 Causes of death of 78 coronary subjects

Causes	Number of subjects
Coronary heart disease (variously listed on death certificates as myocardial infarction, coronary thrombosis, coronary artery disease, ventricular fibrillation, coronary insufficiency, acute circulatory failure, arteriosclerotic heart disease)	67
Paroxysmal atrial tachycardia	1
Ischemic cerebrovascular disease	5
Thrombotic (2)	
Hemorrhagic (3)	
Pulmonary embolism	1
Congestive heart failure	1
Lobar pneumonia	1
Laennec's cirrhosis	1
Carcinoma (right maxillary and ethmoid sinuses)	1

Figure 3.1 Yearly death rate expressed as percentage of surviving coronary patients

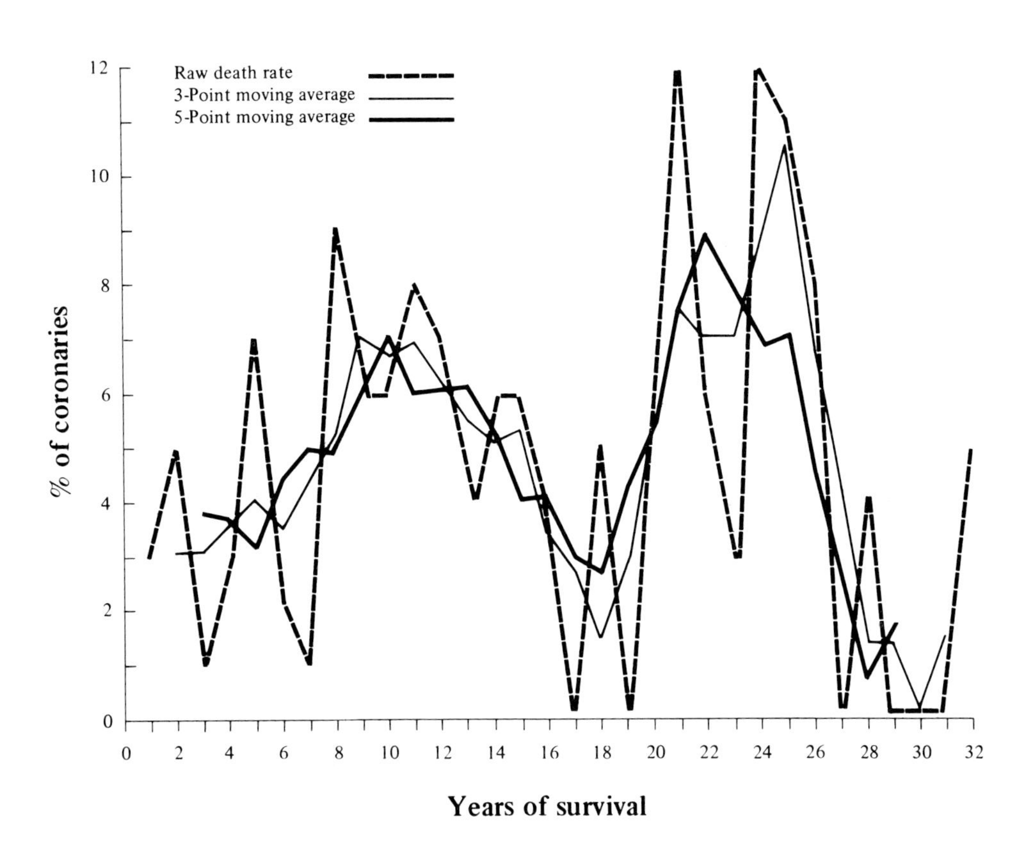

Table 3.6 Post-coronary survival of 78 deceased coronary group members in five-year intervals

Years of survival	Number in group	Average age at onset	Average age at death
0-5	17 (21.8%)	36.94	40.00
6-10	20 (25.6%)	34.70	43.10
11-15	16 (20.5%)	37.00	50.50
16-20	6 (7.7%)	36.33	53.16
21-25	15 (19.2%)	36.40	59.13
26-30	3 (3.8%)	37.00	63.66
31-35	1 (1.8%)	32.00	63.00

Table 3.7 Cumulative per cent mortality in various studies

Year study began	Group	Number	5	10	15	20	25
					Years		
1947	Gertler and White	100	17	37	53	60	78
1940	Weiss	211	40	63	–	–	–
1932	Cole et al.	285	33	56	89	–	–
1926	Richards et al.	162	50	69	86	95	97
1943	Zukel	598	30	49	62	–	–

– no data available

Source: M. M. Weiss, "Ten Year Prognosis of Acute Myocardial Infarction," *Am. J. Med. Sci.* 231: 9-12, 1956; D. R. Cole et al., "The Long-Term Prognosis Following Myocardial Infarction and Some Factors Which Affected It," *Circulation* 9(3): 321-334, 1954; D. W. Richards et al., "A Completed Twenty-five Year Follow-Up Study of 200 Patients with Myocardial Infarction," *J. Chron. Dis.* 4(4): 415-422, 1956; W. J. Zukel et al., "Survival Following First Diagnosis of Coronary Heart Disease," *Am. Heart J.* 78(2): 159-170, 1969.

essence "pure coronaries" relatively unaltered by disease entities known to affect the course of C.H.D. Table 3.7 shows the cumulative per cent mortality of our group in comparison with other studies.

Pure comparison is, of course, not possible because the temporal span alone would make a difference in the socio-economic or cultural patterns, which could alter survival periods and death to some degree. Also, no direct comparison can be made from a patient group in one era to a patient group in another era without some degree of compromise. If one casts aside a puristic tendency and employs empiricism to some extent, then the comparison may become somewhat useful and meaningful. The Framingham mortality data based on 188 male myocardial infarction subjects (including immediate mortality) revealed 45 per cent mortality after six years, 57 per cent mortality after 10 years, and 63 per cent mortality after 14 years.[3] In the case of Zukel's study group, mortality statistics were based on immediate mortality as well as long-term mortality in a group of 598 subjects with myocardial infarction, coronary occlusion, and coronary thrombosis.[4] Richards, Bland, and White studied a group of 200 consecutive cases of myocardial infarction with mortality statistics based on 162 subjects surviving at least four weeks.[5]

Weiss followed a group of 211 cases of myocardial infarction that survived at least two months.[6] The same standards were used in the Cole, Singian, and Katz study.[7]

In analyzing the data in Table 3.7, one is impressed with the fact that in the Richards, Bland, and White data the cumulative deaths were 69.7 per cent in the first 10 years as compared to 37.4 per cent in our coronary group. The cumulative deaths between the 10th and the 20th years in the Richards group and the present coronary group were 25.9 per cent and 22.3 per cent, respectively. Finally, the cumulative deaths between the 20th and 30th years were 3.6 per cent and 18.1 per cent, respectively, in the two groups. The general trend here is that there were approximately 47 per cent surviving after 15 years in our cohort as compared to 14 per cent surviving in Richards' study, which began 23 years earlier. The subjects in this earlier study experienced their coronary event before the emphasis was placed on risk factors, anticoagulants, diet, and exercise.

These data strongly suggest that there is a distinct difference in the way coronary disease was treated from 1926-1956 and 1941-1971, and that the chances of an individual surviving 10 years after recovering from the initial episode is approximately 50 per cent. These conclusions are strengthened by the observation that in both eras there was virtually no difference in death rates during the 10th to 20th years. This could be interpreted as meaning that once the patient survived for 10 years, the death rate remained constant at approximately 2.5 per cent per year. The death rate beyond that time is not comparable because in the earlier study there were virtually 5 per cent surviving after 20 years versus 40 per cent in the present study.

It is interesting to note that individuals who recovered from a heart attack and did not have hypertension, diabetes mellitus, or hypo- or hyperthyroidism increased their chances of surviving more than 10 years. These observations should not be misconstrued and a false conclusion drawn that the absence of hypertension, diabetes mellitus, and hypo- or hyperthyroidism prevents coronary heart disease. This statement is based purely on survival data of a group free of these diseases who have recovered from an initial episode, and it does not have any true bearing on incidence rates for all types of myocardial infarction. It is of further interest that nearly half the present series survived more than 15 years, whereas in the older series (Cole et al. and Richards et al.) the survival rate was less than 10 per cent for 15 years. The Framingham series as well as the Zukel series show one-third of their groups surviving after 15 years; the Framingham data is based solely on myocardial infarction, while Zukel's group includes coronary occlusion, coronary thrombosis, and myocardial infarction.

Another factor appears to manifest itself in the survival pattern of our group, which, while not apparent in the raw data plotted on a yearly basis, becomes more so with the 3- and 5-point moving averages of mortality. The mortality distribution appears to be bimodal with the first mode at 10 years and the second mode at 20 years. The question one asks is, why is there this bimodal distribution of mortality? (See Figure 3.1.)

An analysis of the various parameters employed in this study did not reveal any concrete reasons for the distribution except that the groups differ significantly in age.

Survival in relation to age

The survival period for the coronary and control groups was also evaluated in terms of the differences in the pattern or rate of survival between those who experienced their initial episode prior to age 35 and those who experienced their initial episode after age 35 (see Table 3.8).

The survival ratios in Table 3.9 accentuate the trends and differences in the young and old coronary and control groups and are compared to U.S. life table survival statistics. There is a gradual increase in the differences in the survival ratios in both the older life table group (40 years) and the older control group (≥36 years) when compared to the older coronary group between the initial study period and the 25-year follow-up. There are four times as many nondiseased persons at the end of the 25 years as there are persons with C.H.D. The same order of difference, that is, 2.6:1.0, occurs in the younger group when the survival ratio in the young life table group (30 years) and the younger controls (≤35 years) is compared to the survival rate in the young C.H.D. group (≤35 years).

During the first 20-year follow-up period, one would have expected some differences in the survival ratios between the old life table, control, and coronary groups and

Table 3.8 Per cent survival in young and old coronary and control groups as compared to U.S. life table statistics for all causes

Group	Years: 5	10	15	20	25
Life tables–age 30	99	98	96	93	89
Life tables–age 40	98	95	91	85	77
Control group–≤35 years	98	97	97	92	92
Control group–≥36 years	100	96	94	84	80
Coronary group–≤35 years	88	63	46	44	34
Coronary group–≥36 years	79	64	47	38	19

Source: Life table statistics computed by the Statistical Bureau of the Metropolitan Life Insurance Company from data of the National Center for Health Statistics.

the young life table, control, and coronary groups. This was not so, as may be observed from Table 3.9 where the ratios are virtually the same at 2.1 or 2.2, after 20 years. There is, however, a dramatic change in the survival ratios between the 20th and 25th year of observation where there is a greater ratio of survivors in both the older life table and control survivors with respect to the older coronary group—that is, a ratio of 4.0 to 1.0. In other words, there were four times as many survivors in the older healthy groups as there were in the older coronary group. Similarly, in the younger life table and control survivors there were proportionally fewer deaths than in the younger coronary groups, as is indicated by the ratio of 2.6 to 1.0.

The reasons for this difference during this period (that is, 20-25 years) are not readily apparent. One could conclude that in the older age categories, the individuals have reached the age of 55-plus where demise from C.H.D. and stroke reaches its peak incidence. Thus, the younger individuals (life table, control, and even C.H.D. groups) would be approaching the age of peak incidence, whereas the older individuals would have already reached it. The differences, therefore, in survival ratios could be accounted for by the fact that, in the older C.H.D. groups, the death rate, which is governed by the

Table 3.9 Survival ratios of young and old control, coronary, and life table groups

Years followed	Life table age 40	Control group age ≥36	Life table age 30	Control group age ≤35	Coronary group age ≤35	Life table age 30
	Coronary group age ≥36		Coronary group age ≤35		Coronary group age ≥36	Life table age 40
5	1.2:1	1.3:1	1.1:1	1.1:1	1.1:1	1:1
10	1.5:1	1.5:1	1.6:1	1.5:1	1:1	1:1
15	1.9:1	2:1	2.1:1	1:1	1:1	1:1
20	2.2:1	2.2:1	2.1:1	2.1:1	1.2:1	1.1:1
25	4:1	4.2:1	2.6:1	2.7:1	1.8:1	1.2:1

Figure 3.2 Comparison of survival in young and old coronary and control groups as compared to young and old U.S. life table statistics for all causes

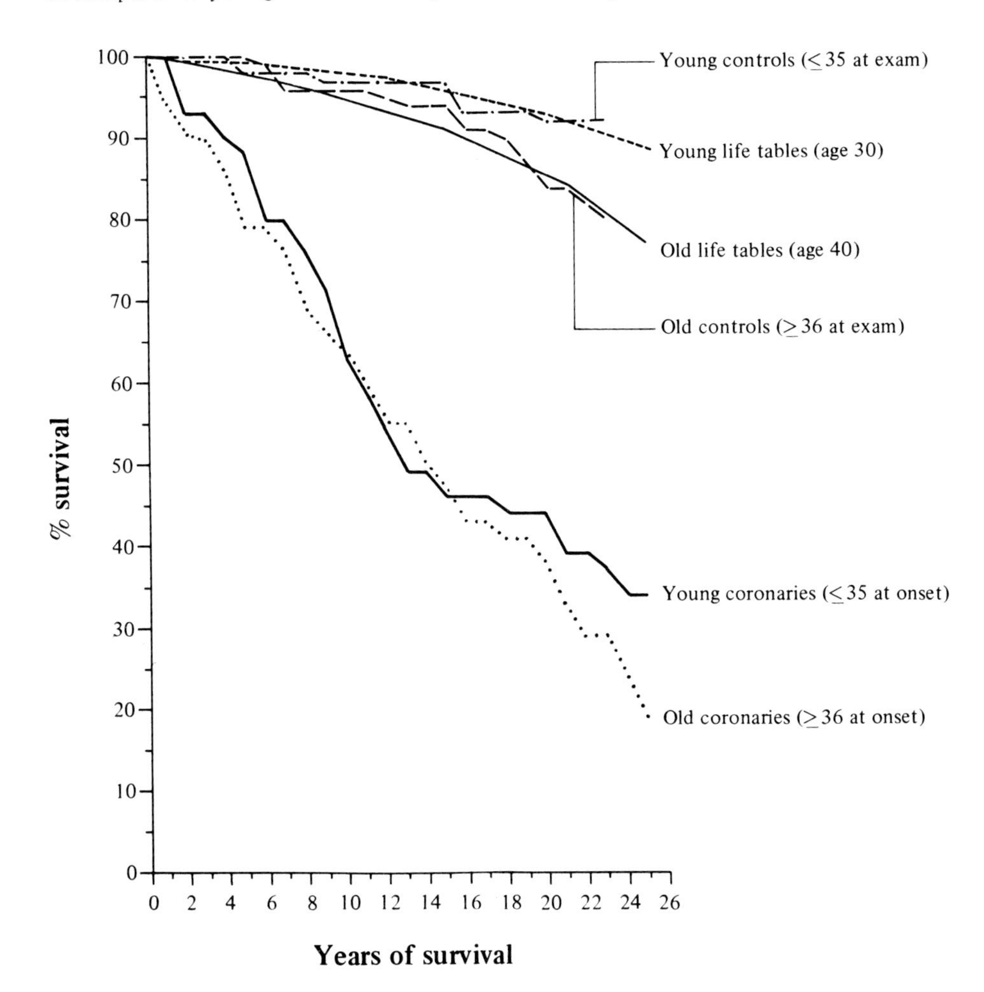

superimposition of the normal death rates, would also be greater in the older C.H.D. group than in the younger C.H.D. group.

Figure 3.2 is the plotting of (a) the general survival patterns of the healthy control group less than and greater than 35 years at the time of the examination, (b) U.S. life table survival based on males aged 30 and 40 years, and (c) survival patterns of the C.H.D. group less than 36 years old at the time of their coronary attacks.

The graph gives the survival rate in percentages after 5, 10, 15, 20, and 25 years for each of these groups.

Survival in the control group

Of the 146 original controls, 100 were factory workers and 46 were executives. A

Table 3.10 Breakdown of survival data for coronary and control groups

	Coronary	Control (factory workers)	Control (executives)
Original number*	100	100	46
Survivors	21 (21%)	89 (89%)	35 (76%)
Deceased	78 (78%)	10 (10%)	11 (24%)
Mean age at death	48.7	53.4	60.2
Mean age of survivors	58.6	58.3	64.3

*One coronary subject and one factory worker control were lost to follow-up.

significant difference ($p<.01$) in the survival pattern of these two groups was found.

There were 10 deaths among the factory worker controls. Three of the control subjects died of coronary heart disease, one of hypertensive arteriosclerotic heart disease, two of ischemic cerebrovascular disease, one each of cirrhosis of the liver and an aortic aneurysm, one of aortic stenosis and pulmonary edema, and one by accidental car death. The average age of the surviving individuals was 58.3 years. The average age of those who died was 53.4 years.

The 11 deaths among the executive control patients occurred at the average age of 60 years. The average age of the survivors was 64.3 years. It is noteworthy that 10 per cent of the factory employes died (that is, those who were doing work that would not be classified as sedentary), whereas 24 per cent of the executives died. This group was composed of executives whose jobs were more sedentary and involved decision making and perhaps a higher caloric intake as well. Interestingly, three of the 11 executives who died succumbed to bronchogenic carcinoma, which may have been related to excessive cigarette smoking. Four died of coronary heart disease, and one each of hypertension, ischemic cerebrovascular disease, esophageal carcinoma, and mesenteric thrombosis. The data support the previously published data from other observers.[8]

The breakdown of survival data for the executive and factory control workers compared to the coronary group is given in Table 3.10.

Clinical Findings at Initial and Follow-Up Examinations

Electrocardiographic findings

Using the three standard limb leads, three unipolar limb leads (AVR, AVL, AVF), and six unipolar precordial leads (V 1 to V 6), evidence of infarction was demonstrable in every case, including one of 10 years' follow-up and another of 21 years' follow-up. This 100 per cent electrocardiographic confirmation is not surprising because in this study the only cases selected were those that had an absolutely certain diagnosis. There were 54 cases of anterior or anteroapical infarction, as evidenced by QRS-wave, ST-segment, and T-wave changes in standard limb leads 1 and/or 2, AVL, and the precordial leads. There were 40 cases of inferior or inferolateral infarctions, as shown by alterations of QRS-ST-T complexes in standard limb leads 2 and/or 3 and lead AVF. In the majority of individuals examined, the whole septum was involved to some extent. Six cases presented the electrocardiographic picture of both anterior and posterior infarctions. The results of these records, which were made at the time of our examination and not during the acute coronary episodes, are summarized in Table 3.11.

Table 3.11 Electrocardiographic findings in the original 100 patients (97 male and 3 female)

	Number of patients
Distribution of myocardial infarction	
Anterior or anteroapical site of infarction	54
Posterior or posterolateral site	40
Both sites	6
Disturbances of rhythm	
Normal sinus rhythm	93
Sinus tachycardia	3
Sinus bradycardia	3
Premature contractions	1
Paroxysmal tachycardia	0
Atrial fibrillation or flutter	0
Conduction defects	
AV block–partial	2
AV block–complete	0
Right bundle branch block	3
Left bundle branch block	2
Other impaired intraventricular conduction	2
No conduction defects	91
Axis deviation	
Left ventricular hypertrophy	11
Left axis deviation	14
Right ventricular hypertrophy	0
Right axis deviation	3
No axis deviation	72

Permission to reproduce granted by Harvard University Press and M. M. Gertler, P. D. White, *Coronary Heart Disease in Young Adults* (Cambridge: Harvard University Press, 1954), p. 16.

Electrocardiograms were also taken on the 20 surviving subjects at the follow-up examination. The ECG had returned to normal in three cases (each had experienced one episode only). In two patients, each of whom experienced only one episode, there was no definite abnormality in the ECG. The summary of ECG findings is found in Table 3.12. Table 3.13 summarizes the electrocardiographic findings for 112 control subjects for the 1971 follow-up examination.

The electrocardiographic findings of the controls in 1971 with and without C.H.D. are compared with the surviving coronary group in Table 3.14.

The tests for significance revealed that there were (a) significant differences between the surviving controls and surviving coronaries (X^2=24.02, $p<.001$) and (b) significant differences between controls without C.H.D. and surviving coronaries (X^2=27.17, $p<.001$).

The ECG findings revealed once again that the ECG can be normal in the presence of coronary heart disease. The question may therefore be asked, should not the stress electrocardiogram be employed to detect the presence of occult or covert C.H.D.? Since the evidence for this manner of testing is becoming very convincing, the stress electrocardiogram should be so used.

Table 3.12 Electrocardiographic findings in 20 surviving coronary cases–1971

Number of patients	Description	Number of episodes
3	Normal	1
2	No definite abnormality	1
3	Healed anteroseptal infarction	1
1	Right ventricular hypertrophy	3
6	Posterior myocardial infarction (one with left posterior hemiblock)	4 patients with this reading had at least 2 attacks each; 2 patients had 1 attack each
2	Anterior myocardial infarction (one with left anterior hemiblock)	1
1	Right bundle branch block	1
1	Nonspecific diagnostic pattern	1
1	Left bundle branch block with anteroseptal and inferior infarction and left ventricular hypertrophy	1

Table 3.13 Electrocardiographic findings in 112 control subjects–1971 follow-up

Description	Number of patients
Normal	91
Abnormal	18
Atrial flutter-fibrillation	3
Myocardial infarction	10
Healed anteroseptal (1)	
M.I. posterior (1)	
M.I. anterior (8)	
Sinus bradycardia	1
Premature ventricular contractions	1
Right bundle branch block	2
Left bundle branch block	1
Borderline	3
Isoelectric–T waves	1
ST segment depressed	1
Hypokalemia	1

Table 3.14 Breakdown of normal and abnormal electrocardiographic findings in control and coronary groups

	Normal	Abnormal	Total
Surviving C.H.D. group	6	14	20
Surviving controls	94*	18	112
Controls with C.H.D.	9	5	14
Controls without C.H.D.	85	13	98

*Three borderline-ECG controls are included in this total.

Fasting blood sugar

The subject of fasting blood sugar and diabetes mellitus will be considered more fully in Chapter X, but there is evidence to support the contention that abnormalities are a contributory risk factor in C.H.D., ischemic thrombotic cerebrovascular disease, and, to some extent, intermittent claudication. Because of this, fasting blood sugar was measured in the control and coronary groups. In 1971, significant differences ($p<.05$) in fasting glucose levels were found between the 99 controls who did not experience an acute episode and the 14 controls who did. The controls with C.H.D. had a mean level of 124.6 mg per cent compared with the controls without C.H.D., who had a mean level of 103.6 mg per cent.

Blood counts

There were no significant differences among the various groups in their hematocrit, hemoglobin, or sedimentation rates, although hematocrit and sedimentation rates were slightly higher in the coronary group.

The 1949 data on 18 of the surviving coronary cases showed a significantly lower mean white blood count ($p<.05$) than the 1949 white blood count of the 62 expired coronaries for whom we had this information (that is, 8,839 for the surviving group and 10,544 for the deceased group). The importance of these findings is confirmed by a recent study indicating that total leukocyte (white cell) count is significantly related to the future development of myocardial infarction.[9]

Our results do not confirm several reports in which elevated hematocrits were found in patients with C.H.D.[10] However, the data in these groups were scanty.

Symptomatology in the surviving coronary group

In the 1971 follow-up it was found that the majority of the surviving coronary patients still experienced angina pectoris. It is interesting to note that only two patients had hypertension. There were three cases of intermittent claudication, and the remaining illnesses appeared to be what one might expect to see in any population of similar age (see Table 3.15).

Blood groups

The association of diseases with certain blood groups has been studied. Jick and others demonstrated that there is a paucity of blood group O in cases of venous thromboembolism.[11] The evidence is supported by the fact that individuals with type O blood have lower levels of antihemophilic globulin (factor VIII), which would favor bleeding. Indeed, the great proportion of bleeding in peptic ulcers occurs in individuals with type O blood.

Pursuing this line of reasoning, Nefzger, Hrubec, and Chalmers in 1969 examined individuals with C.H.D. to determine the blood type distribution.[12] The distribution turned out to be similar to what we observed in our study (see Table 3.16). The Framingham Study's blood type distribution is shown in Table 3.17, along with prevalence, incidence, and mortality rates for C.H.D.[13] They found a significantly lower incidence of nonfatal C.H.D. in the O group, compared to the A group. It should be noted, however, that the C.H.D. groups were composed of not only myocardial infarction patients but coronary-insufficiency and angina-pectoris patients as well. The summary of

Table 3.15 Symptomatology in the surviving coronary group of 21 patients

	Number of patients
Angina pectoris	14
Dyspnea	6
Dizziness	6
Intermittent claudication	3
Hypertension	2
Premature ventricular contraction	2
Emphysema	1
Chronic bronchitis	1
Asthma	1
Prostatitis	3
Hemorrhoids	4
Cancer	2
Abdominal aneurysm	2
Ulcer	4
Gallbladder disease	2
Ulcerative colitis	1
Renal calculi	1
Hiatus hernia	1
Arthritis	2

Table 3.16 Comparison of blood type distribution in two study groups, in per cent

	Nefzger et al.		Gertler, White et al.	
	M.I. (n=816)	Controls (n=6, 611)	M.I. (n=84)	Controls (n=146)
A	48.4	40.6	44	35
B	11.0	10.9	16.6	14.4
AB	4.4	3.8	4.8	2.7
O	36.2	44.7	34.5	48

Source: M. D. Nefzger, Z. Hrubec, and T. C. Chalmers, "Venous Thromboembolism and Blood-Group," *Lancet* 1:887, 1969.

Table 3.17 Distribution, prevalence, and incidence rate in Framingham men according to blood type

Group	Number	Per cent	C.H.D. alive prevalence rate/1,000	4 years' C.H.D. incidence rate/1,000	
				Alive	Deceased
A	704	38.3	82	51	13
B	202	11.0	109	45	0
AB	66	3.6	76	0	0
O	865	47.1	82	27	15

Source: R. J. Havlik, M. Feinleib, R. J. Garrison, and W. B. Kannel, "Blood Groups and Coronary Heart Disease," *Lancet* 2:269-270, 1969.

Table 3.18 Blood group classification and Rh factor in coronary and control groups*

	A	B	AB	O	Total	Rh+	Rh−
Coronary cases	37	14	4	29	84	73	9
Surviving coronary cases	10	0	1	9	20	15	5
Deceased coronary cases	27	14	3	20	64	57	3
Controls	51	21	4	70	146	117	29
Controls without C.H.D.	41	16	3	63	123	99	24
Controls with C.H.D.	10	5	1	7	23	18	5

*Rh factor is not available for all subjects.

our own data on blood type classification is found in Table 3.18 for both control and coronary groups.

There have been published reports relating the level of serum lipids to blood types.[14] It appears that individuals with type A blood are the most susceptible to hyperlipidemia, followed by type B, AB, and O in descending order. The blood group data from this study were matched against the levels of various lipids and uric acid. The results are summarized for the various categories in Table 3.19.

It was generally noted that serum cholesterol was higher in those individuals with type A blood, independent of their control or coronary group classification. These results generally confirm those reported in the literature. The only group that showed a statistically significant difference between blood types for cholesterol was the total coronary group for the 1949 determination. The lipid phosphorus values did not differ significantly, though the uric acid level was significantly higher in the controls who developed C.H.D. and had blood type A than in those with blood type O.

Rh factor

Although very little has been published on Rh factors and their relationship to C.H.D., our data show that there was a distinct difference between the surviving C.H.D. and the deceased C.H.D. groups with regard to Rh groups ($p<.05$). The surviving C.H.D. group had a larger number of negative-Rh-factor individuals than the deceased coronary group. The ratio of Rh-positive to Rh-negative individuals in the total C.H.D. group was 8.1:1. Among the C.H.D. survivors the ratio was 3.0:1; among the C.H.D. deceased the ratio was 19.0:1.

These differences did not extend to the control group. The ratio of Rh-positive to Rh-negative individuals in the total control group was 4.0:1. In the control group without C.H.D., the ratio was 4.1:1. Among the controls with C.H.D. the ratio was 3.6:1. Among the deceased controls with C.H.D. the ratio was 2:1.

Blood pressure

Hypertension is now considered to be a primary risk factor in coronary heart disease, though the data appear to be based merely on the association between blood pressure readings and the incidence and morbidity of C.H.D. A mere association does not warrant the assumption of a causal relationship. This statement is strengthened by the observations of Perera and Pickering, who demonstrated statistically significant longevity

Table 3.19 Mean cholesterol, uric acid, and lipid phosphorus in the coronary and control groups by blood type

Group	1949			1971		
	Cholesterol	Uric acid	Lipid phosphorus	Cholesterol	Uric acid	Lipid phosphorus
Surviving coronaries						
Type A (10)	270 ± 61	4.5 ± 1.1	12.2 ± 2.5	255.7 ± 42	6.1 ± 8	10.8 ± 1.6
Type B (0)	–	–	–	–	–	–
Type AB (1)	294	4.3	10.6	243	6.2	9.5
Type O (9)	223.8 ± 46	4.8 ± 1.1	11.0 ± 1.2	268.7 ± 56	6.2 ± 1.1	11.6 ± 1.9
Controls with C.H.D.						
Type A (10)	236.7 ± 22	4.5 ± 1.0	12.4 ± 1.1	264.7 ± 43.6	6.7 ± 0.6	11.0 ± 1.4
Type B (5)	222.2 ± 25	4.5 ± 1.5	11.7 ± 1.9	243.5 ± 33.2	6.7 ± 0.3	10.2 ± 2.8
Type AB (1)	187	3.8	9.1	–	–	–
Type O (7)	241.1 ± 49.3	4.8 ± 0.9	12.6 ± 1.0	200.5 ± 56.2	4.6 ± 1.8	9.0 ± 1.7
All coronaries						
Type A (37)	299.3 ± 75.2	4.9 ± 1.2	12.8 ± 2.3	–	–	–
Type B (14)	280.3 ± 89.3	5.2 ± 1.0	12.4 ± 2.2	–	–	–
Type AB (4)	294.0 ± 32.9	5.4 ± 1.4	13.2 ± 2.4	–	–	–
Type O (29)	265.8 ± 52.8	5.2 ± 1.1	12.2 ± 1.8	–	–	–
Deceased coronaries						
Type A (27)	310.0 ± 79.8	5.1 ± 1.2	13.1 ± 2.2	–	–	–
Type B (14)	280.3 ± 89.5	5.2 ± 1.0	12.4 ± 2.2	–	–	–
Type AB (3)	294.0 ± 40.3	5.8 ± 1.4	14.6 ± 1.0	–	–	–
Type O (20)	284.0 ± 55.5	5.4 ± 1.1	12.8 ± 2.0	–	–	–
All controls						
Type A (51)	231.3 ± 43.6	4.8 ± 0.9	12.2 ± 1.6	239.9 ± 39.3	5.9 ± 1.3	10.3 ± 1.4
Type B (21)	221.5 ± 32.0	4.5 ± 0.9	11.6 ± 1.6	218.2 ± 34.8	5.9 ± 0.7	9.7 ± 1.5
Type AB (4)	213.5 ± 43.3	4.5 ± 1.0	11.3 ± 3.0	179.3 ± 22.5	5.9 ± 0.9	9.0 ± 1.7
Type O (70)	221.1 ± 43.3	4.7 ± 0.8	12.1 ± 1.8	239.9 ± 37.2	6.0 ± 1.3	10.1 ± 2.0
Controls without C.H.D.						
Type A (41)	230.0 ± 47.4	4.9 ± 1.0	12.2 ± 1.7	234.6 ± 38.3	5.7 ± 1.4	10.2 ± 1.4
Type B (16)	221.2 ± 34.0	4.5 ± 0.6	11.6 ± 1.5	214.0 ± 35.1	5.8 ± 0.7	9.6 ± 1.1
Type AB (3)	222.3 ± 66.0	4.7 ± 1.1	12.1 ± 3.2	192.0 ± 7.1	5.5 ± 0.8	9.7 ± 2.0
Type O (63)	219.0 ± 42.6	4.7 ± 0.8	12.0 ± 1.9	226.0 ± 35.4	6.1 ± 1.3	10.2 ± 2.0

in patients with hypertension.[15] Furthermore, more recent reports by Brunner, Laragh, and Baer lend specific support to these clinical observations.[16] They demonstrated that there was not a single instance of acute C.H.D. or stroke in hypertensives who had low renin values, despite the fact that left ventricular enlargement was present in equal proportion in both the low and high renin groups (20 and 22 per cent respectively). The low renin group comprised 27 per cent of the population. Another incongruity in these data is that this cohort was comprised of 42 per cent blacks, an ethnic group in which hypertension is supposedly associated in large proportions, not one of whom experienced coronary vascular disease.

Brunner, Laragh, and Baer reported eight cases of C.H.D. in a group of 219 patients, all of whom had normal or high renin excretion. The question that arises here is, why were there no instances of C.H.D. in the low renin group, only two in the high renin group, and six in the normal renin group? The distribution certainly points to factors other than elevated blood pressure as the cause of C.H.D. This question is now being considered by a national study that is attempting to resolve the importance of hypertension, smoking, and cholesterol as individual and/or multiple risk factors for C.H.D. Perhaps such a study will shed some light on why it is reported that 600,000 die annually from C.H.D., while 200,000 die from ischemic cerebrovascular disease, and only 25,000 die from hypertensive heart disease or hypertensive renal disease.

The data in Figure 3.3 were obtained from the present coronary group and published earlier.[17] They emphasize the importance of separating hypertension from serum cholesterol levels in assessing their influence on risk rates.

The present groups of coronary patients and controls were selected on the basis of absence of hypertension. They were also selected prior to the age of 40, thus giving hypertension ample time to develop by 1972. This was in accordance with the thesis that hypertension and atherosclerosis are not independent of each other. In 1949, the highest systolic blood pressure in the coronary group was 160 mm Hg, the highest diastolic pressure was 108 mm Hg, with the average for the group being 123/81. In the 1971 follow-up, the highest systolic blood pressure in the surviving coronary group was 200 mm Hg; the highest diastolic pressure was 98 mm Hg. Only two coronary patients were reported as being hypertensive.

In 1949, the mean blood pressure of the coronary subjects was not significantly different from the controls, which was expected. The same results were observed in the 1971 follow-up data, when the various surviving groups were compared. Table 3.20 summarizes the blood pressure data.

The one significant difference observed was between the controls who did not develop C.H.D. and the original C.H.D. group in 1949 for diastolic pressure only. It should be noted, however, that the diastolic pressure did not attain abnormal levels.

Delta values of blood pressure

The delta values are an indication of the changes in blood pressure in the various groups between 1949 and 1972. These values are tabulated in Table 3.21.

In 110 controls from whom blood pressure data were obtained in 1949 and 1972, there was a significant rise of 14.41 and 5.25 mm Hg in the systolic and diastolic pressures, respectively. Similar significant changes were observed in the surviving controls

Figure 3.3 The interrelationships of changing blood pressure values and changing serum cholesterol levels on the risk of coronary artery disease in healthy men. Note the effects of serum cholesterol levels alone (A) and the effects of blood pressure values alone (B).

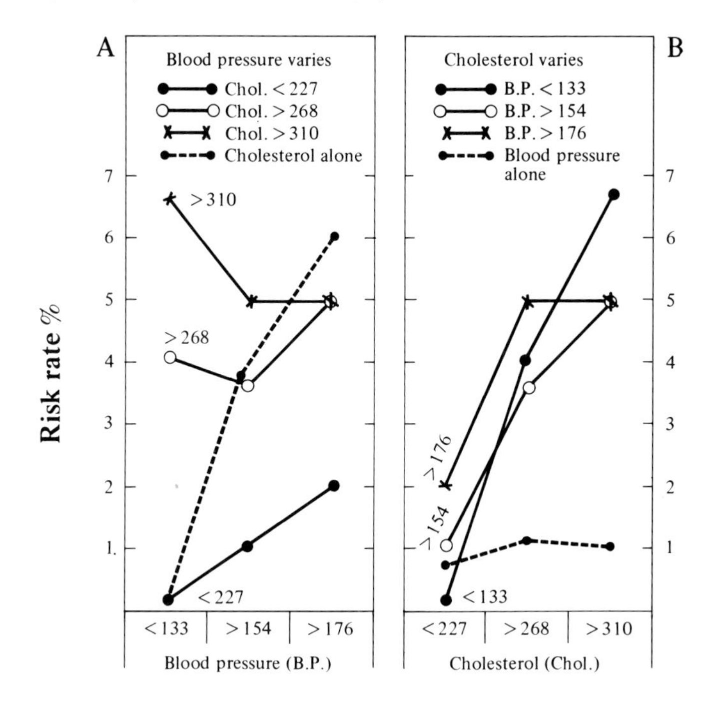

Permission to reproduce granted by The New York Academy of Sciences and M. M. Gertler, H. Whiter, "Individual Differences Relating to Coronary Artery Disease," *Ann. New York Acad. Sci.* 134: 1041-1045, 1966.

who did not develop C.H.D. and in the 13 surviving controls who subsequently developed C.H.D. Interestingly, the surviving coronaries had the smallest rise in systolic and diastolic blood pressure, or 8.44 and 2.39 mm Hg respectively. These differences were not significant.

In spite of the significant differences in the delta values, neither the average systolic nor average diastolic blood pressure rose above the accepted limits of normal. Thus, the element of hypertension did not arise on an average basis.

Arcus senilis

Arcus senilis was found in five of the 20 surviving coronary cases and 12 of the 115 controls examined in 1971. Arcus senilis was originally considered to be related to cholesterol metabolism, and Boas stated that the incidence of arcus senilis increased with hypercholesterolemia.[18] This concept was later questioned, and additional evidence was presented that did not support Boas' thesis. When the degree of arcus senilis was matched

Table 3.20 Mean blood pressure of coronary and control groups in 1949 and 1971

	1949		1971	
	Mean	Number	Mean	Number
All coronary cases	123/81	96	135/84	19
All controls	120/78	146	133/83	110
Controls with C.H.D.	120/80	23	137/84	13
Controls without C.H.D.	120/78	123	132/82	97
Surviving coronary group	123/81	21	135/84	19
Expired coronary group	124/81	78	–	–

Table 3.21 Delta values of blood pressure for coronary and control groups

	Number	Mean ± S.D.	t	p<
Surviving coronaries	19	sys. 8.44 ± 17.88	2.00	ns
		dias. 2.39 ± 12.18	0.83	ns
Surviving controls	110	sys. 14.41 ± 19.94	7.58	.001
		dias. 5.25 ± 12.15	4.53	.001
Controls without C.H.D.	97	sys. 13.02 ± 19.18	6.68	.001
		dias. 4.71 ± 12.48	3.72	.001
Controls with C.H.D.	13	sys. 24.77 ± 23.13	3.86	.01
		dias. 9.23 ± 8.59	3.87	.01

with cholesterol levels and lipoprotein patterns, no correlation was found. This appears to confirm other observations as well.[19]

Cigarette smoking

Cigarette smoking is now considered a primary risk factor for C.H.D.[20] This statement is based on several lines of evidence that show a direct relationship between the incidence of C.H.D. and increasing cigarette smoking, although there are a few investigators who do not subscribe to this conclusion.[21] We should like to add the evidence that we have accumulated on this subject.

In the first issue of this monograph the following conclusions were made: (a) There were more smokers in the coronary group than in the control group. (b) Of the smokers in both groups, those in the coronary group smoked more cigarettes daily.

In the 1971 follow-up, smoking data were analyzed only in terms of the number of cigarettes smoked, since it was found that cigar and pipe smoking were minimal. The data were divided into three categories: those controls who never smoked, those who used to smoke, and those who still smoked.

The data revealed that in the surviving coronary group one patient never smoked, six of the 10 survivors who used to smoke had averaged 33.3 cigarettes a day, while nine of the 10 who presently smoked averaged 25.3 cigarettes a day. Thus, there were patients who had recovered from C.H.D. and who still smoked at least a pack of cigarettes daily.

Within the control population, 24 did not smoke, 30 of the 47 who used to smoke had averaged 28.6 cigarettes a day, while 38 of the controls who still smoked averaged 29.9 cigarettes daily. Of the 14 controls who experienced C.H.D., two never smoked, four of the six who previously smoked had averaged 27.5 cigarettes daily, while five of the six who presently smoked averaged 26.4 cigarettes daily.

There were no significant differences found between either of the groups, though the question of weight change in relation to smoking was raised in our follow-up data. It was found that in the control group, nonsmokers had gained an average of 6.1 pounds, former smokers 12.3 pounds, and present smokers almost no weight, or 0.66 pounds. One could speculate whether the gain in weight by past smokers was not, perhaps, more harmful to the coronary arteries than the continuation of cigarette smoking.

The basic question about the relationship between cigarette smoking and C.H.D. revolves around the influence of nonsmoking and the cessation of smoking on the disease. Does the cessation of smoking alone cause a reduced risk of C.H.D. in both primary and secondary prevention programs? Do nonsmokers have a lesser risk of getting heart disease than smokers? Another question to consider is whether the cessation of smoking or the absence of cigarette smoking will reduce the risk of C.H.D. in the presence of hypercholesterolemia, hyperuricemia, hypertension, diabetes mellitus, positive family history, and overweight. The effect of cigarette withdrawal cannot be assessed in terms of its real or relative value in reducing the risk rate of C.H.D. until it has been studied as an individual variable. Such studies are being considered at the present time. There is no doubt that cigarette smoking does affect the incidence of cancer of the lung and lung diseases in general. Whether the effects of smoking on C.H.D. are direct or indirect cannot be answered at this time.

It is also interesting to note that there was a direct relationship between cigarette smoking and alcohol consumption in our study group. It was observed that those who never smoked drank the least, while those who presently smoked drank the most. This offers additional evidence that the causal relationship or association between smoking and C.H.D. demands further investigation.

Alcoholic intake

There have been reports that excessive intake of alcoholic beverages contributes to C.H.D.[22] The scanty evidence suggests that alcoholic intake in excessive amounts accounts for weight gain, which, it is thought, produces a series of changes such as hypercholesterolemia, hypertriglyceridemia, and eventually, atherosclerotic heart disease. There is another line of evidence that considers alcohol as a carbohydrate; when taken in excessive amounts, it alone results in hypertriglyceridemia. The evidence for both these views is far from conclusive. In 1949, the coronary group ingested more liquor in the form of whiskey and gin than the unmatched control group. In total quantities, however, the unmatched group ingested more alcoholic beverages of all kinds (mostly beer), or 38 ounces per week compared to the coronaries' 34 ounces.

In the 1971 follow-up, alcoholic intake was broken down and analyzed in three categories: those controls and coronaries who did not drink or just drank socially, those considered moderate drinkers, and those who were heavy drinkers (see Table 3.22).

Table 3.22 Alcoholic intake in coronary and control groups in 1971 follow-up

	None or socially	Moderate	Heavy
Surviving coronaries	8 (38.1%)	10 (47.6%)	3 (14.3%)
Controls	42 (33.6%)	71 (56.8%)	12 (9.6%)
Controls without C.H.D.	35 (31.8%)	65 (59%)	10 (8%)
Controls with C.H.D.	7 (46.6%)	6 (40%)	2 (13.3%)

The chi square analyses did not reveal any significant differences between the groups. Thus, there does not appear to be any direct evidence in our data to link alcoholic intake to C.H.D. There is some indirect evidence that excessive alcoholic intake, through its action on the liver, causes a failure on the part of the liver to conjugate estrogens, which could lead to increased risk of C.H.D. It has been observed that (a) females do not show an increased incidence of C.H.D. until postmenopause, (b) men who have been subjected to bilateral orchiectomy early in life do not experience C.H.D., and (c) experimental animals fed estrogens do not experience the severity of cholesterol arterial deposits that nonestrogen-fed animals experience.

Studies on Salivary Amylase and Oxidation-Reduction Potentials

The classification of lipoproteins into various phenotypes, such as types I to V with several subdivisions, suggests that there is a degree of carbohydrate abnormality in the genesis of coronary heart disease. This observation, coupled with the increased propensity of individuals with diabetes mellitus to develop coronary heart disease, has strengthened the concept that some degree of abnormality is associated with coronary heart disease.

Dextrinizing time

In 1949, the studies on the coronary and control groups concerning the ability of salivary amylase to catabolize starch in the amyloclastic phase of starch digestion as measured by an iodine test suggested that individuals with short dextrinizing time are the most prone to coronary heart disease. An independent survey was also made in 1960. When the values for the two groups were compared in 1949 and 1960, they were significantly different. It was also found that the control group in 1949 and 1960 differed significantly from the additional C.H.D.-prone group studied in 1960. When the values of the C.H.D. and C.H.D.-prone groups were compared, no significant differences existed, as was expected.

In 1971, the dextrinizing times of the three groups were re-evaluated based on the survival data up to that time. There was a near significant difference between the surviving and deceased controls in 1949 and 1960 as well. A significant difference was also found between the control survivors and the C.H.D.-prone group that did not subsequently develop the disease, for 1949 and 1960 values. In addition, there was a near significant difference between the C.H.D.-prone group that did not develop the disease and the C.H.D.-prone group that did develop the disease. The reasons for the barely missed significance in most cases was due, it is believed, to the limited sample size, because the trend for significance was apparent.

Table 3.23 Significant differences in dextrinizing time between control and coronary groups in 1949 and 1960 and coronary-prone group of 1960

Group and year	Number	Mean ± S.E.	t	p<
Control (1949)	12	27.5 ± 5.24		
C.H.D.-prone (1960)	10	13.9 ± 2.25	2.21	.05
Control (1949)	12	27.5 ± 5.24		
C.H.D. (1949)	37	10.8 ± 1.10	4.74	.001
Control (1949)	12	27.5 ± 5.24		
C.H.D. (1960)	20	10.3 ± 0.95	4.09	.001
Control (1960)	20	28.1 ± 3.29		
C.H.D.-prone (1960)	10	13.9 ± 2.25	2.87	.01
Control (1960)	20	28.1 ± 3.29		
C.H.D. (1949)	37	10.8 ± 1.10	6.09	.001
Control (1960)	20	28.1 ± 3.29		
C.H.D. (1960)	20	10.3 ± 0.95	5.21	.001

Table 3.24 1971 follow-up of significant differences in dextrinizing time between control and coronary groups of 1949 and 1960 and coronary-prone group of 1960

Group and year	Number	Mean ± S.E.	t	p<
Control survivors (1949)	9	28.5 ± 4.80		
Control deceased (1949)	2	6.5 ± 0.50	2.06	.10
Control survivors (1949)	9	28.5 ± 4.80		
C.H.D.-prone w/o C.H.D. (1960)	8	16.0 ± 2.59	2.25	.05
Control survivors (1960)	18	28.5 ± 3.43		
C.H.D.-prone w/o C.H.D. (1960)	8	16.0 ± 2.59	2.32	.05
C.H.D.-prone w/o C.H.D. (1960)	8	16.0 ± 2.59		
C.H.D. survivors (1960)	17	10.5 ± 1.03	2.58	.05

From these studies it was concluded that salivary amylase was helpful in classifying individuals with covert C.H.D. as well as in distinguishing between coronary and control groups (see Tables 3.23 and 3.24).

Oxidation-reduction potentials

The oxidation-reduction potential is a quantitative measurement of the ability of substances to donate or accept electrons. Thus, this measurement is an indication of free energy changes in oxidation-reduction reactions.

In 1949, salivary oxidation-reduction potential was measured in 66 members of the original coronary group and 66 control group members of roughly similar age, ethnic origin, body build, and mouth condition, drawn from the matched control group. The

Table 3.25 Tests for significant differences in salivary oxidation-reduction potential between coronary group of 66 males and control group of 53 males free of C.H.D.

Time	Controls free of C.H.D.		Coronary group		t	p<
	Number	Mean ± S.E.	Number	Mean ± S.E.		
15 sec.	53	290.6 ± 6.29	66	271.1 ± 5.28	2.40	.01
1 min.	48	263.0 ± 6.89	60	245.7 ± 7.82	1.61	ns
2 min.	49	235.1 ± 7.72	61	217.9 ± 9.11	1.40	ns
3 min.	45	207.3 ± 10.62	57	193.1 ± 11.60	0.88	ns
4 min.	43	201.0 ± 10.83	60	169.5 ± 13.20	1.74	ns
5 min.	51	179.9 ± 11.72	62	114.5 ± 15.19	1.78	ns
10 min.	53	101.5 ± 18.54	60	34.7 ± 26.45	2.02	.05
15 min.	49	44.7 ± 24.68	60	−48.1 ± 31.63	2.23	.05
20 min.	49	−17.2 ± 30.62	56	−121.3 ± 34.00	2.25	.05
25 min.	50	−58.7 ± 32.92	56	−169.0 ± 37.31	2.19	.05
30 min.	51	−108.6 ± 34.57	63	−213.1 ± 38.01	1.99	.05

results of these studies, published in the 1954 monograph, revealed several noteworthy differences. A significant difference was noted at the 15-second and 15-, 20-, 25-, and 30-minute intervals between the two groups. The general trend over the complete test period was downward, with the coronary heart disease group being distinguished by having lower potential than the control group at all intervals. With elapsed time the differences tended to be larger, revealing that the over-all rate of change was greater in this group. These differences may be attributed to the degree of concentration of various inorganic ions and/or combinations of enzymes or coenzymes that are present in the saliva of the coronary and healthy males.

The most noteworthy finding of the follow-up study was the increase in the degree and number of significant differences between the two groups when those controls who had subsequently developed heart disease were screened out (see Table 3.25). When the controls who had developed C.H.D. were compared to the original coronary group, no significant differences were noted. This finding was expected, and it supports the contention that there is little biochemical difference, as measured by these parameters, between an individual who is incubating C.H.D. and one who already has C.H.D.

Summary

The follow-up study revealed many interesting clinical findings. There were 21 living members of the original coronary group with an average survival period of approximately 24 years since their first coronary episode. The highest death rate from C.H.D. occurred among the patients in managerial positions in both the coronary and control groups. Season, once again, did not appear to greatly influence the acute disease occurrences.

There were 17 individuals who experienced three or more acute episodes before their demise. The period of survival for these patients was between 11.6 and 18.5 years. It was determined, however, that survival period was unrelated to the age at onset, based on the fact that the ages at onset were virtually the same. The mortality in our series of patients was also found to be less than in other series (see Table 3.7). Perhaps the selection of the C.H.D. group, the treatment they received, and the present-day treatment (which appears to normalize the risks somewhat through secondary prevention) accounted for this. A bimodal distribution of survival was also noted in our group (one mode at 10 and the other at 22 years), but statistical analyses could not determine the reasons, if any, for this occurrence.

U.S. life table statistics for all causes were compared to our coronary and control groups in reference to age, revealing a precipitous drop in the survival rate in both young and old members of the C.H.D. group for the first 15 years. An increasing death rate was noted in the older members of the coronary group along with a less precipitous fall in the younger members. The survival of both younger and older controls paralleled comparable life table statistics.

The follow-up electrocardiograms revealed once again that the ECG can be normal in the presence of coronary heart disease, although there was a significant difference between the control and coronary groups in terms of abnormal ECG response. This points up the value of using the more definitive, sensitive stress electrocardiogram.

Among the other clinical differences noted were a higher fasting blood sugar in the coronary group and a higher white blood count in the surviving coronary cases as opposed to the expired coronaries for the 1949 determination. Also noted was a significantly greater number of Rh-negative patients in the surviving coronary group and a greater number of Rh-positive subjects in the deceased coronary group. Generally speaking, a higher serum cholesterol level was found in coronary patients with type A blood than in the other blood groups. The distribution of blood types in this series was similar in proportion to other series compared—that is, approximately 45 per cent of the C.H.D. group had type A blood, 16 per cent had type B blood, 5 per cent had type AB blood, and 35 per cent had type O blood. Blood pressure values were not significantly different in the coronary and control groups, although both groups had experienced a significant increase in blood pressure over the last 25 years, but not to hypertensive levels. As for cigarette smoking, no significant differences were found between the study groups. Nor were any differences revealed for alcoholic intake between the two groups.

Salivary amylase and oxidation-reduction potential studies were made to investigate the relationship between carbohydrate metabolism and coronary heart disease. It was demonstrated that individuals who had rapid dextrinizing times were most prone to coronary heart disease. The follow-up data emphasized the importance of salivary dextrinizing times in that differences were found between the control and C.H.D.-prone groups that did not develop the disease subsequently. This was in addition to there being a near significant difference in the C.H.D.-prone group between those who did and those who did not develop C.H.D. Studies on salivary redox potentials were also very revealing in that they demonstrated no significant difference between the controls who developed the disease and the coronary group. Another interesting observation was that when the controls who developed the disease were removed from the control series, the significant differences increased between the "purer" control group and the coronary group.

References

1 E. A. Hooton, Personal communication.

2 W. M. Yater, A. H. Traum, W. G. Brown et al., "Coronary Artery Disease in Men Eighteen Years of Age," *Am. Heart J.* 36: 334-372, 1948; W. H. Gordon, E. F. Bland, and P. D. White, "Coronary Artery Disease Analyzed Post-Mortem With Special Reference to the Influence of Economic Status and Sex," *Am. Heart J.* 17: 10-14, 1939; L. E. Hinkle Jr., "Occupation, Education and Coronary Heart Disease," *Science* 161: 238-246, 1968.

3 W. B. Kannel and T. Gordon, eds., *The Framingham Study: An Epidemiologic Investigation of Cardiovascular Disease,* Section 25 (Washington, D.C.: U.S. Government Printing Office, Sept., 1970) Table 4B.

4 W. J. Zukel, B. M. Cohen, T. W. Mattingly, and Z. Hrubec, "Survival Following First Diagnosis of Coronary Heart Disease," *Am. Heart J.* 78(2): 159-170, 1969.

5 D. W. Richards, E. F. Bland, and P. D. White, "A Completed Twenty-five Year Follow-Up Study of 200 Patients With Myocardial Infarction," *J. Chron. Dis.* 4(4): 415-422, 1956.

6 M. M. Weiss, "Ten Year Prognosis of Acute Myocardial Infarction," *Am. J. Med. Sci.* 231: 9-12, 1956.

7 D. R. Cole, E. B. Singian, and G. N. Katz, "The Long-Term Prognosis Following Myocardial Infarction and Some Factors Which Affected It," *Circulation* 9(3): 321-334, 1954.

8 S. L. Syme, M. M. Hyman, and P. E. Enterline, "Some Social and Cultural Factors Associated With the Occurrence of Coronary Heart Disease," *J. Chron. Dis.* 17: 277-289; A. Keys, ed., "Coronary Heart Disease in Seven Countries," *Circulation* 41(4): 1-211, 1970.

9 G. D. Friedman, A. L. Klatsky, and A. B. Siegelaub, "Leukocyte Count as Predictor of Myocardial Infarction," *New Eng. J. Med.* 290: 1275-1278, 1974.

10 G. E. Burch and N. P. Depasquale, "The Hematocrit in Patients With Myocardial Infarction," *JAMA* 180: 63-65, 1962.

11 H. Jick, B. Westerholm, M. P. Vessey et al., "Venous Thromboembolic Disease and ABO Blood Type," *Lancet* 1: 539-542, 1969; B. Bronte-Stewart, M. C. Botha, and L. H. Krut, "ABO Blood Groups in Relation to Ischemic Heart Disease," *Brit. Med. J.* 1: 1646-1650, 1962.

12 M. D. Nefzger, Z. Hrubec, and T. C. Chalmers, "Venous Thromboembolism and Blood-Group," *Lancet* 1: 887, 1969.

13 R. J. Havlik, M. Feinleib, R. J. Garrison, and W. B. Kannel, "Blood Groups and Coronary Heart Disease," *Lancet* 2: 269-270, 1969.

14 L. Hagerup, P. F. Hansen, and F. Skov, "Serum-Cholesterol, Serum-Triglycerides and ABO Blood Groups in a Population of 50-Year-Old Danish Men and Women," *Amer. J. Epid.* 95(2): 99-103, 1972.

15 G. A. Perera, "Relation of Blood Pressure Lability to Prognosis in Hypertensive Vascular Disease," *J. Chron. Dis.* 1: 121-126, 1955; G. W. Pickering, *High Blood Pressure,* 2nd ed. (London: J. and A. Churchill Limited, 1968), pp. 299-312.

16 H. P. Brunner, J. H. Laragh, L. Baer et al., "Essential Hypertension: Renin and Aldosterone Heart Attack and Stroke," *New Eng. J. Med.* 286(9): 441-499, 1972.

17 M. M. Gertler and H. Whiter, "Individual Differences Relating to Coronary Artery Disease," *Ann. N.Y. Acad. Sci.* 134: 1041-1045, 1965.

18 E. P. Boas, "Arcus Senilis and Arteriosclerosis," *J. Mt. Sinai Hosp.* 13: 79-83, 1945.

19 S. M. Garn and M. M. Gertler, "Arcus Senilis and Serum Cholesterol Levels in the Aleut," *New Eng. J. Med.* 242: 283-285, 1950; O. Paul, M. H. Lepper, W. H. Phelan et al., "A Longitudinal Study of Coronary Heart Disease," *Circulation* 28: 20-31, 1963.

20 J. Stamler, *Lectures on Preventive Cardiology* (New York: Grune and Stratton, 1967), pp. 139-143; F. H. Epstein, "The Epidemiology of Coronary Heart Disease—a Review," *J. Chron. Dis.* 18: 735-774, 1965; J. T. Doyle, T. R. Dawber, W. B. Kannel et al., "The Relationship of Cigarette Smoking to Coronary Heart Disease," *JAMA* 190: 886-890, 1964.

21 Syme et al., "Some Social and Cultural Factors," 277-289; Keys, "Coronary Heart Disease," 1-211; C. C. Seltzer, "Cigarettes and Heart Disease," *New Eng. J. Med.* 284: 557-558, 1971.

22 J. H. Mitchell and L. S. Cohen, "Alcohol and the Heart," *Mod. Concepts Cardiovasc. Dis.* 39(7): 109-113, 1970; L. Gould and R. F. Gomprecht, "Alcoholic Heart Disease," *Geriatrics* 25: 130-132, 1970.

IV Family Incidence: The Role of Heredity

The concept of heredity has changed considerably since the days of Mendelian genetics. Today's concept is more far-reaching and penetrating, since it encompasses not only the overt characteristics that were originally studied, such as blue eyes, but also the enzyme systems that are controlled by the gene. Thus, molecular biology is in reality the basis of understanding the overt characteristics of blue eyes as well as the intricate workings of enzyme deficiency diseases, such as Lesch-Nyhan, where the deficiency of hypoxanthine-guanine phosphoribosyl transferase is responsible for a series of biochemical events reflected in clinical symptomatology. Accordingly, if a single gene is lacking, which in turn fails to generate the necessary enzyme to complete a series of so-called normal events, then one should be able to reason that similar events can occur in far more complicated diseases such as coronary heart disease.

The above preamble does not mitigate against the past clinical observations that coronary heart diseases occur more frequently in parents, siblings, and close relatives of the propositus patients. Rather, it clarifies our understanding of the observations. It has been demonstrated that all of the so-called risk factors do have a hereditary basis; thus, hypercholesterolemia,[1] hyperuricemia,[2] type II, IV, and other lipoprotein abnormalities occur in certain families.[3] It is reasonable to suggest, therefore, that less overt combinations of these factors that are responsible for the overt manifestations of the disease do exist in patients with coronary heart disease.

A study made in Denmark has a strong bearing on this point. Kornerup studied 331 members of four families with familial hypercholesterolemia. He observed that the average age of coronary death in 41 hypercholesterolemic men was 56 years as compared with 70 years in nonhypercholesterolemic men.[4] The findings were similar in women.

Some authors believe that a genetic predisposition may be enhanced by environmental tendencies, such as a diet high in saturated fats in a hypercholesterolemic, hyperlipidemic individual.[5] Such observations coincide with the biochemical concept of enzyme induction, which is defined as the de novo production of an enzyme protein by specific substances (inducers) in the growth environment. Thus, in human beings, excessive inducers could be responsible for enzyme induction with consequences unknown at this time.

Clinical cardiologists have observed coronary heart disease in families since the disease was first diagnosed.[6] Only in recent years, however, has this observation been documented. The documentation has gone even further in that several authors have noted an increase in the disease in fathers, mothers, and siblings of the propositi.[7] The relatively higher incidence in the families cannot be attributed solely to the inheritance of the known risk factors or to the environmental aspects. There are doubtless many other factors involved that are presently not considered as primary risk factors, such as coagulation factors. This point is emphasized in a study on the incidence of coronary heart disease in monozygotic and dizygotic twins. The influence of heredity is suggested by a higher concordance rate of C.H.D. among monozygotic twins compared to dizygotic twin pairs, or 9.2, 2.0 and 21.7, 6.1, respectively, for the age ranges of 40-60 years and 60-80 years.[8]

Family Mortality and Average Length of Life at Initial Interview

Data pertaining to the physical status of parents and siblings were obtained from the coronary and control groups in an effort to determine the number of deaths and instances of coronary heart disease in their families.

The frequency and cause of death among parents of the coronary and control groups were studied at the initial interview. It was found that the proportion of parents living at that time was higher in the unmatched control group than in the coronary group. Of the mothers, 73 per cent were alive in the control group as opposed to 58 per cent in the coronary group. Similarly, 45 per cent of the fathers of the control group members were alive as compared with 32 per cent of the coronary group's fathers. These differences are statistically significant, and it was therefore concluded that mortality was higher among the parents of the patient group.

To determine whether the differences in mortality could be attributed to a difference in age distribution in the two groups of parents, the ages of the surviving parents at that time were compared. No statistically significant difference could be found, however, ruling out this possibility. It was also noted that the average age at death of the parents of the coronary group was slightly lower than in the control group, although this difference was not statistically significant.

When the causes of death were compared, it was found that both the mothers and fathers of the coronary group showed a larger proportion of deaths due to cardiovascular disorders of all kinds than the control group's parents (51.3 per cent and 35.9 per cent of the mothers, and 64.6 per cent and 46.2 per cent of the fathers, respectively). The same order of difference was found among fathers who died specifically of diseases of the coronary arteries, that is, 37.1 per cent and 18.5 per cent. This difference is significant. Practically no difference was found in the percentages of death from diseases of the coronary arteries between the mothers of the two groups.

It must be kept in mind that there is room for error when information stems from a source that is subject to bias or error by the individual. It is altogether possible for a patient to give a "retrospective" diagnosis, assuming the parent died of the same disorder that afflicts the patient himself. It should be pointed out, however, that the proportions of death due to "old age," unknown cause, accident, and so forth are comparable in both groups.[9]

Frequency and cause of death among siblings

At the time of the original interview, 20 per cent of the control siblings and 15 per cent of the coronary siblings had died. The causes of death, however, showed a marked difference between the two groups. The deceased siblings of the coronary group showed an excess of cardiovascular disorders; that is, 27.6 per cent of the coronary siblings died of various cardiovascular disorders compared with 8.2 per cent of the deceased siblings of the control group. This difference is statistically significant, much of the difference having been due to the higher coronary heart disease rate among siblings of the young coronary patients. Five of the 58 deceased siblings of the coronary group had died from coronary heart disease as compared to one in 98 in the control group. When diseases of infancy were compared in the siblings, it was found that 45 per cent of the deaths in the control group could be attributed to this cause as compared to 26 per cent in the coronary group. The reasons for this difference are not readily apparent.

Findings on heredity

The genealogies of the coronary and control groups were analyzed to determine whether the mode of inheritance followed any simple genetic model. At the time of the original study, it was found that in 73 of the 100 coronary cases, neither parent exhibited the disease. In only three cases did both parents have the disease. Eight and six-tenths per cent of the siblings of the coronary patients experienced coronary heart disease, whereas only 1 per cent of the siblings of the unmatched controls had coronary heart disease. This difference is statistically significant. For 131 of the 146 controls, neither parent was said to have had coronary heart disease. In no case were both parents of controls affected. Three mothers in the control group had a history of the disease—almost the same number as in the patient group. Only 14 fathers of the 146 controls were affected, as compared with 26 fathers of the coronary group of 100. The incidence of the disease, then, was significantly greater in the parents of the patients (15 per cent) than in the parents of the control group (5.8 per cent).

The genealogies failed to show a spectacular number of family members with coronary heart disease. Few genealogies replete with heart disease were found, and genealogies with many affected siblings were absent, though this may well be attributed in part to the relatively low age of both the coronary and control groups at the time of the original study. From the data, it would appear to be highly unlikely that the disorder was inherited as a simple Mendelian dominant or as a dominant covert in the female. The possibility that the disorder was inherited as a Mendelian recessive was checked further, and it was found to be highly unlikely. The most definite statement that can be made is that the disorder runs in families, and is possibly a multifactor condition with at least one dominant factor.

Follow-Up Results

Method

The follow-up data on family history were accumulated in the following manners: (a) direct interview of the surviving coronary disease patients and the surviving members of the control group, and (b) correspondence with spouses, siblings, sons, daughters, parents, relatives, and physicians of the deceased members of the coronary and control groups. In the event that no updated information could be obtained, the 1949 data were used. If the parents of the coronary and control subjects were free of heart disease at the time of the original study, and no new information could be obtained, the old data were omitted. We thus avoided making assumptions about whether the relatives were still free of coronary heart disease.

Results of the follow-up

The family history of coronary heart disease in 1949 forms an interesting base with which to compare the family histories as they existed in 1971. These data reveal that in 1949, when the coronary heart disease group and the control group were virtually the same age (an average of 38 years old), the degree of coronary heart disease in the parents of the control group was much lower, as can be seen in Table 4.1. However, by 1971, the incidence of coronary heart disease in the fathers of the control group was numerically greater than in the fathers of the coronary heart disease group, although not greater in terms of per cent. The difference between the two groups did not attain statistical significance. The percentage of mothers who had developed C.H.D. was about the same in both groups, and the same can be said of both parents developing C.H.D. These data indicate that C.H.D. had a natural increase in the parents of both groups as the parents became older. However, the degree of genetic penetrance to their offspring was greater in the case of the coronary heart disease group. Similar reports were derived from Thomas and Cohen's study.[10]

When family histories of the expired coronary group were compared with the surviving coronary group, no significant differences were observed. The ratio between afflicted and unafflicted parents was essentially the same between the two groups. There were also no significant differences observed between the coronary disease group and the control group with regard to subsequent coronary heart disease, as was expected. These results are not surprising because essentially the comparisons were made between groups of a certain homogeneity; that is, the coronary groups, whether surviving or deceased, did possess essentially similar hereditary patterns. This is emphasized in the nonsignificant differences in the observed comparisons between the members of the control group who subsequently developed coronary heart disease and the entire coronary group.

Table 4.2 is probably the most important table because it demonstrates significant differences in the hereditary findings between the siblings of the entire coronary heart disease group and the siblings of the members of the control group who did not develop heart disease. It shows that coronary heart disease may be transmitted via hereditary mechanisms.

No significant differences were found in the immediate family histories between the members of the control group who subsequently developed coronary heart disease and

Table 4.1 Family history of coronary heart disease in parents of the coronary and control groups in 1949 and 1971 follow-up, in per cent

	Coronary group		Control group	
	1949	1971	1949	1971
Fathers only	26	43.6	9.6	36.3
Mothers only	4	28.7	2.0	29.8
Both parents	3	13.9	0	17.7

Table 4.2 Tests for significant differences in family history of coronary heart disease between coronary group and control group without C.H.D.–1971 follow-up

	Coronary group (100)		Controls without C.H.D. (123)			
	Number	Per cent	Number	Per cent	X^2	p<
Father	44	44	43	39.4	.2158	ns
Mother	27	27	31	28.4	.0147	ns
Brother	43	43	15	13.7	20.353	.001
Sister	21	21	6	5.5	9.613	.001

members of the control group who did not develop coronary heart disease, although the chi square approached significance, or 2.84 in the father category.

It is noteworthy that in the original 1949 data, there were more than twice as many fathers with coronary heart disease in the coronary group as there were in the control group (26 per cent versus 9.6 per cent). These data generally bear out the results of a related study by Ibrahim and his colleagues on the presence of coronary risk factors in 92 high school students and their fathers.[11] The authors found positive correlations between the fathers and students for cholesterol, systolic blood pressure, and ponderal index. Furthermore, the fathers with coronary heart disease, ST- and T-wave abnormalities, and high blood pressure could be identified by singling out those students with observed high levels of the variables measured.

Summary of findings on race

The details of the findings on race have been published elsewhere. In essence, the findings of this survey on ethnic origin revealed that nearly all the ethnic groups on the East Coast were represented in this series. The proportion of individuals ultimately derived from the Near East, however, was approximately 29 per cent, which is well in excess of the general proportions in the United States and the urban Boston area (the home of 70 per cent of the patients).

It has been questioned by previous investigators whether an excess of Jewish patients was due to a higher incidence of coronary heart disease within that group. Since the actual number of cases studied was not great, specific conclusions pertaining to the general American population cannot be made.

Summary

There is an accumulation of data that lends credence to the view that hypercholesterolemia, hyperuricemia, and type II and IV hyperlipoproteinemia occur in some families more frequently than in others. Thus, factors associated with increased risk of coronary heart disease may be genetically transmitted, at least in certain families. With this in mind, we studied the history of coronary heart disease in the families of the control and coronary groups.

At the time of the original study it was clearly demonstrated not only that mortality was greater among parents of the coronary group but also that deaths due to cardiovascular causes were also greater. In the coronary group, 37.1 per cent of the fathers and 9.8 per cent of the mothers died from disease of the coronary arteries as compared to 18.5 per cent and 7.7 per cent, respectively, in the control group. A similar trend was found when mortality among the siblings was analyzed. In the coronary group, 27.6 per cent of sibling deaths were due to cardiovascular disease; in the control group, 8.2 per cent.

At the conclusion of the follow-up, almost 25 years later, the incidence of coronary heart disease among the fathers of the coronary group was still greater than among fathers of the control group, although the incidence among mothers of the control group had slightly surpassed that for mothers of the coronary group. Among siblings there was a very significant difference in the incidence of heart disease; 43 per cent of the brothers and 21 per cent of the sisters of the coronary patients had a history of heart disease, as opposed to 13.7 per cent and 5.5 per cent, respectively, in the control group.

On the basis of the evidence accumulated here, it is reasonable to conclude that coronary heart disease is more likely to occur in the individual whose mother, father, or siblings have experienced the disease. Follow-up studies have indicated the presence of a hereditary process that gives more than a 50 per cent chance of penetrance of a cluster of genes responsible for coronary heart disease.[12]

References

1 D. Adlersberg, "Inborn Errors of Lipid Metabolism: Clinical, Genetic and Chemical Aspects, "*Arch. Path.* 60: 481-492, 1955.

2 C. J. Smyth, C. W. Cotterman, and R. H. Freyberg, "The Genetics of Gout and Hyperuricemia: An Analysis of Nineteen Families," *J. Clin. Invest.* 27: 749-759, 1948; J. H. Talbott, "Gout," *J. Chron. Dis.* 1:338-345, 1955.

3 D. S. Fredrickson and R. I. Levy, "Familial Hyperlipoproteinemia," in *The Metabolic Basis of Inherited Disease*, 3rd ed., J. B. Stanbury, J. B. Wyngaarden, and D. S. Fredrickson, eds. (New York: McGraw-Hill, 1972) pp. 545, 614.

4 V. Kornerup, *Familiaer Hypercholesterolaemi og Xanthomatose* (Kolding, Denmark: Konrad Jorgensen, 1948), pp. 1-211.

5 Report by the Central Committee for Medical and Community Program of the American Heart Association, "Dietary Fat and Its Relation to Heart Attacks and Strokes," *JAMA* 175: 389-391, 1961; A. Antonis and I. Bersohn, "The Influence of Diet on Serum-Triglycerides," *Lancet* 1: 3-9, 1961.

6 J. H. Musser and J. C. Barton, "The Familial Tendency of Coronary Disease," *Am. Heart J.* 7: 45-51, 1931; R. R. Gates, *Human Genetics* (New York: Macmillan Co., 1946), pp. 730-742. F. H. Epstein, "Hereditary Aspects of Coronary Heart Disease," *Am. Heart J.* 67(4): 445-456, 1964; J. Jensen, D. H. Blankenhorn, and V. Kornerup, "Coronary Disease in Familial Hypercholesterolemia," *Circulation* 36: 77-82, 1967; S. Deutscher, L. D. Ostrander, and F. H. Epstein, "Familial Factors in Premature Coronary Heart Disease—a Preliminary Report From the Tecumseh Community Health Study," *Amer. J. Epid.* 91: 233-237, 1970; S. Deutscher, F. H. Epstein, and J. B. Keller, "Relationship Between Familial Aggregation of Coronary Heart Disease and Risk Factors in the General Population," *Amer. J. Epid.* 89: 510-520, 1969.

7 L. N. Katz, J. Stamler, and R. P. Pick, *Nutrition and Atherosclerosis* (Philadelphia: Lea and Febiger, 1958), pp. 1-146; J. Stamler, *Lectures on Preventive Cardiology* (New York: Grune and Stratton, 1967), pp. 152-154; Inter-Society Commission for Heart Disease Resources, Atherosclerosis Study Group and Epidemiology Study Group, "Primary Prevention of the Atherosclerotic Diseases," *Circulation* 42: A55, 1970; F. H. Epstein, "Risk Factors in Coronary Heart Disease—Environmental and Hereditary Influences," *Israel J. Med. Sci.* 3: 594-607, 1967; E. A. Murphy, "Some Difficulties in the Investigation of Genetic Factors in Coronary Artery Disease," *Canad. Med. Ass. J.* 97: 1182-1192, 1967; C. M. Bloor, "Hereditary Aspects of Myocardial Infarction," *Circulation* 40 (Suppl. 4): 130-135, 1969.

8 R. Cederlof, L. Friberg, and E. Johnson, "Hereditary Factors and Angina Pectoris," *Arch. Environ. Health* 14: 397-400, 1967.
9 M. M. Gertler, P. D. White et al. *Coronary Heart Disease in Young Adults.* The Commonwealth Fund (Cambridge: Harvard University Press, 1954), p. 26.
10 C. B. Thomas and B. H. Cohen, "The Familial Occurrence of Hypertension and Coronary Artery Disease With Observations Concerning Obesity and Diabetes," *Ann. Int. Med.* 42: 90-127, 1955.
11 M. A. Ibrahim, W. Pinsky, M. Kohn et al., "Coronary Heart Disease: Screening by Familial Aggregation," *Arch. Environ. Health* 16: 235-240, 1968.
12 R. A. Rohde, "The Chromosomes in Heart Disease: Clinical and Cytogenetic Studies of 68 Cases," *Circulation* 34: 484-502, 1966; K. H. Ehlers and M. A. Engle, "Familial Congenital Heart Disease: Genetic and Environmental Factors," *Circulation* 34: 504-516, 1966; J. German, K. H. Ehlers, and M. A. Engle, "Familial Congenital Heart Disease II: Chromosomal Studies," *Circulation* 34: 517-523, 1966.

V Anthropometric and Morphological Appraisal of Physique

The original study on body form and weight in the C.H.D. and control groups proved to be a powerful impetus for other groups to confirm, extend, and modify the conclusions published in the 1954 version of this text. The over-all conclusions suggest that body build is a strong factor in the assessment of C.H.D. and may be considered a risk factor. This chapter contains a review of our work on this subject, as well as that of other investigators; an analysis of follow-up data on the coronary and control groups; and a discussion of the literature dealing with anthropometric and morphological characteristics related to coronary heart disease.

Historical Background

Many early surveys of coronary heart disease dealt with physique in such undefined terms as "obese" and "overweight." A greater percentage of obese and overweight individuals showed up in the coronary groups studied than in the healthy groups.[1] But Yater et al., reporting on a very extensive Army series, noted that the men who ultimately died after experiencing verified coronary atherosclerosis with infarction were overweight at the time of induction but not at the time of death.[2] This important observation questioned the role of weight per se in the etiology of coronary heart disease and raised the problem of whether weight reduction constituted any real preventive therapy. Moritz and Zamcheck similarly showed that Army men who died after coronary occlusion were no heavier than Army men who died accidental deaths, although both groups were overweight according to norms based on inductee statistics.[3] This explained some findings while, at the same time, questioning the validity of earlier studies. It was concluded, however, that overweight alone did not seem to be a factor. The main problem with these earlier studies was the great latitude in the definitions of the terms "obese" and "overweight."

The physique factor in heart disease, rather than weight alone, was stressed by other investigators, but the actual description of physique was not yet formulated.[4] Despite the lack of agreement in the studies themselves, most clinicians assumed that fat was an etiological factor in coronary heart disease and they employed weight reduction for therapy. The questions we hoped to answer in the present study were:

1. What physique distribution actually exists among individuals who have heart disease at an early age?
2. Is obesity a prime etiological factor in this disorder?
3. Is there a "coronary" physique type?

The program set up at the time of the original study was designed to investigate (a)

Table 5.1 A list of anthropometric measurements in 97 C.H.D. cases and 146 controls with significant differences

	C.H.D. Mean ± S.E.	Controls Mean ± S.E.	p<
Weight (lb)	170.5 ± 2.3	177.0 ± 2.0	.05
Stature (cm)	171.8 ± 0.6	176.3 ± 0.7	.01
Span (cm)	176.5 ± 0.8	179.6 ± 0.6	.05
Chest length (cm)	21.5 ± 0.2	22.4 ± 0.2	.01
Total face (mm)	121.1 ± 0.6	123.6 ± 0.6	.01
Hand length (mm)	191.2 ± 0.9	193.8 ± 0.6	.05
Shoulder breadth (cm)	39.2 ± 0.2	40.1 ± 0.2	.01
Upper chest depth (cm)	19.5 ± 0.2	18.5 ± 0.2	.01
Wrist depth (mm)	41.1 ± 0.3	39.9 ± 0.2	.01
Bipupillary (mm)	62.8 ± 0.3	65.4 ± 0.3	.01

Table 5.2 A list of anthropometric indices in 97 C.H.D. cases and 146 unmatched controls with significant differences

Index	C.H.D. Mean ± S.E.	Control group Mean ± S.E.	p<
Ponderal	12.25 ± .06	12.43 ± .05	.05
Thoracic	76.8 ± .6	74.4 ± .5	.01
Relative span	102.9 ± .4	101.8 ± .2	.05
Waist-hip	99.9 ± .7	98.3 ± .4	Borderline
Eye-face	92.2 ± .7	94.1 ± .6	.05
Hand breadth	46.3 ± .5	45.3 ± .3	Borderline

Table 5.3 Distribution of ponderal indices in C.H.D. group of 97 males and unmatched control group of 146 males

Ponderal index	Coronary group		Control group	
(ht/$\sqrt[3]{\text{weight}}$)	Number	Per cent	Number	Per cent
10.0-10.9	0	0.0	1	0.7
11.0-11.4	4	4.1	4	2.7
11.5-11.9	24	24.8	29	19.8
12.0-12.4	39	40.3	46	31.5
12.5-12.9	20	20.7	47	32.2
13.0-13.4	8	8.2	13	8.9
13.5-13.9	2	2.0	4	2.7
14.0-14.4	0	0.0	2	1.4

anthropometric characteristics determined by standard measurements; (b) gross morphological characteristics of each coronary patient in terms of physique, habitus, or body build; and (c) weight in relation to both accepted standards and to the weight of a control group, as well as weight-height ratios. In all, 24 body measurements were made to test the alleged obesity of coronary heart disease patients as well as indicate the general physique or body type.

Anthropometric Measurements and Indices

Measurements were taken at the time of the original study that could determine whether differences were (a) general, (b) concentrated in the thoracic trunk, or (c) peripheral. To test specifically for obesity, measurements of waist breadth and hip breadth were taken on the assumption that abdominal flaccidity is the best single measure of obesity.

The measurements taken of the thoracic trunk were chest depth (upper and lower), chest breadth, and chest length (sternum-ensiform). There were four measurements of the peripheral region: hand length, hand breadth, wrist depth, and wrist breadth. Ten measurements of the head and face were taken: bipupillary, nose length, nose breadth, upper face length, total face length, biocular, bizygomatic, bigonial, head breadth, and head length.

The indices analyzed were ponderal index, thoracic index, relative span, hip-shoulder index, waist-hip index, upper facial index, eye-face index, nasal index, shoulder index, hand breadth index, wrist breadth index, and cephalic index.

When the measurements and indices of the original coronary and control groups were compared, it was found that the control group, in general, was taller and more linear than the coronary group. The difference was best seen in height, span, total face length, hand length, and chest length. Span is the measurement from fingertip to fingertip when the arms are fully extended. Total face length is a caliper measure of nasion (by projection) to menton. Hand length is the measurement from the third wrist crease to the tip of the index finger, while chest length is measured from the sternal notch to the palpated bony tip of the xiphoid process.

It was also found that while the coronary group had a tendency to be shorter than the controls, they were also significantly broader, as seen in the differences in shoulder breadth (the biacromial measurement taken from the front), upper chest breadth (the distance from the midmanubrium to the spine), wrist depth (a dorsal-ventral measurement at right angles to the forearm), and bipupillary (the interpupillary diameter with eyes relaxed). (See Table 5.1.)

Two of the significant indices were ponderal and thoracic. The ponderal index is a measure of body mass (height divided by the cube root of weight), while the thoracic index is a measure of chest roundness (lower chest depth divided by chest breadth). The differences in the measurements between the two groups well illustrate the evidence that the coronary heart disease group was relatively heavier per foot of stature and showed central distribution of weight (see Table 5.2). The distribution of the two groups, according to the ponderal index, is given in Table 5.3. The other two indices that showed significant differences were relative span (span divided by height multiplied by 100),

Table 5.4 Significant differences in anthropometric variables between surviving coronaries and surviving controls

Variable	Surviving C.H.D. group Number	Mean ± S.D.	Surviving controls Number	Mean ± S.D.	t	p<
Bipupillary	21	62.7 ± 2.5	124	64.9 ± 3.0	3.20	.01
Biocular	21	114.1 ± 4.9	124	108.5 ± 5.3	4.57	.001
Shoulder breadth	21	39.3 ± 1.2	122	40.1 ± 1.6	2.71	.01
Nose breadth	21	37.4 ± 2.9	124	36.1 ± 2.7	2.04	.05
Total face length	21	119.3 ± 5.4	121	122.8 ± 6.5	2.31	.05
Hip-shoulder	21	75.9 ± 3.5	112	74.1 ± 5.3	2.01	.05

Table 5.5 Significant differences in anthropometric variables between deceased and surviving controls

Variable	Deceased controls Number	Mean ± S.D.	Surviving controls Number	Mean ± S.D.	t	p<
Age	21	41.7 ± 5.2	124	36.0 ± 7.0	3.57	.001
Hand breadth	21	87.2 ± 4.1	122	90.7 ± 16.6	2.01	.05

Table 5.6 Significant differences in anthropometric variables between controls who developed C.H.D. and controls who did not develop C.H.D.

Variable	Controls with C.H.D. Number	Mean ± S.D.	Controls without C.H.D. Number	Mean ± S.D.	t	p<
Age	25	41.5 ± 5.6	120	35.9 ± 6.9	3.82	.001
Hand breadth	24	86.6 ± 4.1	119	91.0 ± 16.7	2.51	.01

Table 5.7 Significant differences in anthropometric variables between controls who developed C.H.D. and all coronaries

Variable	Controls with C.H.D. Number	Mean ± S.D.	All coronaries Number	Mean ± S.D.	t	p<
Age	24	41.7 ± 5.6	97	38.4 ± 4.9	2.88	.01
Stature	24	175.1 ± 6.5	97	171.6 ± 6.4	2.40	.05
Upper chest depth	23	18.5 ± 1.4	97	19.5 ± 2.1	2.74	.01
Sternum-ensiform	24	22.5 ± 1.8	96	21.4 ± 1.7	2.74	.01
Bipupillary	24	65.2 ± 3.1	97	62.7 ± 3.4	3.47	.001
Wrist breadth	24	39.3 ± 3.0	97	41.1 ± 3.2	2.39	.05
Biocular	24	108.3 ± 5.2	97	114.1 ± 6.2	4.26	.001
Head length	24	196.6 ± 6.3	97	193.2 ± 7.4	2.09	.05

which gives a measure of relative body weight, and the eye-face index (bipupillary distance divided by upper face length multiplied by 100), which yields a measure of relative eye-face breadth.

Results of the follow-up

In comparing the surviving C.H.D. group with the surviving control group, we were impressed with the ectomorphic similarity of the two groups. The groups were approximately the same height and had the same ponderal index and sternum-ensiform measurements. These characteristics may offer some protection to the individual with C.H.D., which is in keeping with the observation that ectomorphy, or linearity, is less frequently associated with C.H.D. (See *Rating of Physique.*)

The surviving coronary group had greater measurements in nose breadth, hip-shoulder length, and biocular length. The biocular length is the measurement of the distance between the right orbital border and left orbital border at the level of the frontozygomatic suture. The measurements of shoulder breadth, total face length, and bipupillary distance were smaller in the coronary survivors. The total face length and hip-shoulder length were in keeping with the tendency towards ectomorphy in this group, which correlated with their long-term survival (see Table 5.4).

There were no real differences in measurements between the 21 deceased controls and the 124 surviving controls that would account for the differences in survival between the two groups. The only measurements that differentiated these two groups were age and hand breadth, the deceased controls having been older and having had narrower hands. The comparison between the controls who developed C.H.D. (deceased or living) and the 122 non-C.H.D. controls reveals that the C.H.D. controls were older and had narrower hands (see Tables 5.5 and 5.6).

When we studied the controls who subsequently developed C.H.D. and compared them to the entire coronary group, we found several important differences. The controls who developed C.H.D. were older and taller at the time of examination. They also had a longer sternum-ensiform (chest length), a longer head length, and wider bipupillary diameters. In addition, they had narrower upper chest depths, wrist breadths, and biocular diameters. These differences did not offer any leads about survival or occurrence of C.H.D. in these individuals (see Table 5.7).

There is an interesting observation to be made about the differences between the long- and short-term survivors in the C.H.D. group. The short-term survivors—those who lived five years—had a narrower shoulder breadth than those who survived 15 years. This pattern manifested itself in the group surviving 10-15 years. The pattern is not consistent in chest breadth or hip breadth. The other measurements taken do not show as consistent a trend as shoulder breadth in discriminating between the five-year and 10-15-year survival group, although this is lost in the over-15-year survival period (see Table 5.8).

The meaning of this unusual finding—increasing shoulder breadth in the long-term survivors—cannot be readily explained at this time. This unique difference may be related to a higher chest breadth (chest depth ratio), which suggests a less "asthmatic" type chest and, hence, better aeration. Better pulmonary gas exchange may or may not be related to increased C.H.D. survival.[5]

Rating of Physique

A major problem for consideration in this study has not been weight itself but whether, in comparing physical characteristics of the coronary and control groups, the differences or similarities in weight and weight indices might be due to different proportions of constituent tissues. In other words, as indicated previously, the problem has been one of physique rating.

The requirements of this study necessitated a physique rating system marked by the following features:

1. It would follow the concept of morphological constitution—"the principle that the individual's bodily habitus is unchangeable once it is established"[6] —distinguishing between habitus and nurture.
2. It would be age-corrected so that age and nutritional features would not be confused with constitutional differences, nor would one age be a standard for all ages.
3. The individual would be rated numerically and without reference to "types."
4. The ratings would show "useful correlations."

Somatotype method

While the vast majority of physique rating systems (Kretschmer's, Viola's, and others) have employed bipolar or even tripolar typologies (thus necessitating a few "extreme" or "pure" types and a large "mixed" category), the Sheldonian system of somatotyping makes use of three polar extremes only as directions, designating the

Table 5.8 Significant differences in short- and long-term survival in coronary group in relation to anthropometric variables

Variable	<5 Years (N) Mean ± S.D.	5-10 Years (N) Mean ± S.D.	10-15 Years (N) Mean ± S.D.	>15 Years (N) Mean ± S.D.
Shoulder breadth	(14) 37.8 ± 2.45	(19) 38.7 ± 1.85	(17) 39.6 ± 1.38	(47) 39.4 ± 1.49

t-test

Category	t	p<
5 vs. 5-10	1.20	ns
5 vs. 10-15	2.43	.05
5 vs. >15	3.00	.01

Variable	<5 Years (N) Mean ± S.D.	5-10 Years (N) Mean ± S.D.	10-15 Years (N) Mean ± S.D.	>15 Years (N) Mean ± S.D.
Chest breadth	(14) 28.7 ± 3.02	(19) 29.6 ± 2.13	(17) 31.1 ± 1.37	(47) 29.9 ± 1.96

t-test

Category	t	p<
5 vs. 5-10	1.17	ns
5 vs. 10-15	2.93	.01
5 vs. >15	1.76	ns

various combinations, in terms of distance, along the three directions.

To quote Sheldon: "The important aspect of somatotyping is not the number of somatotypes, but the fact that human physiques are measured in terms of three basic components. These components can be scaled against continuous scales, and it is only for purposes of convenience that we divide these scales by means of seven points at equal-appearing intervals."[7] The numerical rating system in the Sheldonian sense avoids typology, though the terminology makes it possible to designate the position of the physique in words as well as in numbers.

The three components that are rated in this system are endomorphy, mesomorphy, and ectomorphy. Endomorphy is the component of softness, roundness, and smoothness, but not necessarily of fat. Mesomorphy is the component of muscularity, bone mass, and angularity of outline and contour. Ectomorphy is the component of linearity, fragility, and elongation. Each individual is given a three-number rating, with each number representing the relative dominance of a physique component. The highest number represents the dominant component, the next highest number the secondary component, and the lowest number the least prominent component.

Methods used in present study

Ratings were established on the basis of standardized photographs, together with weight-height data and the patient's health history. After determining the dominant and secondary components, the numerical ratings were applied. This method of numerical rating–by degree of each physical component–differed from those previously used by noting not only the direction of the physique but also the distance to which the physique extended in that direction. For example, on a sliding scale of 1 to 7 (for which 1 and 7 represent the extremes of any dominance), a person with a rating of 7-1-1 (endomorphy–mesomorphy–ectomorphy) and another person with a rating of 4-3-3 would both be considered dominant endomorphs. Yet there is a major difference between them. There are some cases in which no one component is clearly dominant and others in which two components may be equal, as in the 5-5-1 and 4-4-2 individual. In still other and rarer cases all three components may be about equal, as in a 4-4-4 individual.

In the course of this study it was possible to employ not only the information provided by the immediate appearance of the individual but also all the valuable data provided by the interview and the health history. Naturally, far more data were obtained on the young coronary heart disease patients, who were subjected to intensive interview, than on the controls. However, in the unmatched control group, records were made of the weight at 20-25 years of age, maximum weight, occupation, and athletic interest. Therefore, the final ratings were based on a more detailed knowledge of the individual than momentary appearance alone would have provided. Preliminary sorting was only accomplished after studying all this information according to the somatotype system to see if there was evidence that major differences existed in one component.

Results of the original study

As shown in Table 5.9, there was evidence that the coronary heart disease group and the control group differed in the distribution of their dominant components. The major differences (see Figures 5.1 and 5.2) occurred within the category of dominant

Figure 5.1 Distribution of physiques among 97 young male coronary heart disease patients. In this group the mesomorphs were the most common, while ectomorphs were surprisingly rare.

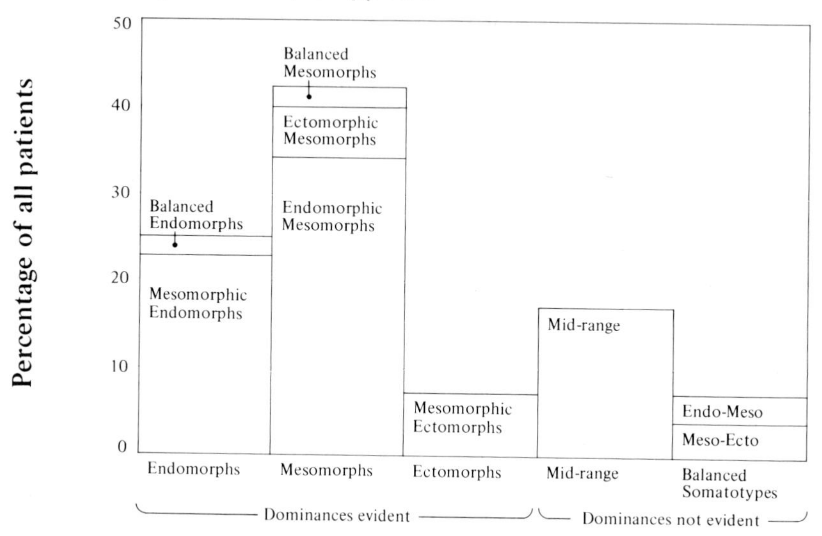

Permission to reproduce granted by Harvard University Press and M. M. Gertler, P. D. White, *Coronary Heart Disease in Young Adults* (Cambridge: Harvard University Press, 1954), p. 56. Copyright 1954 by The Commonwealth Fund.

Figure 5.2 Distribution of physiques among 146 unmatched controls. In this group the endomorphs had a slight predominance.

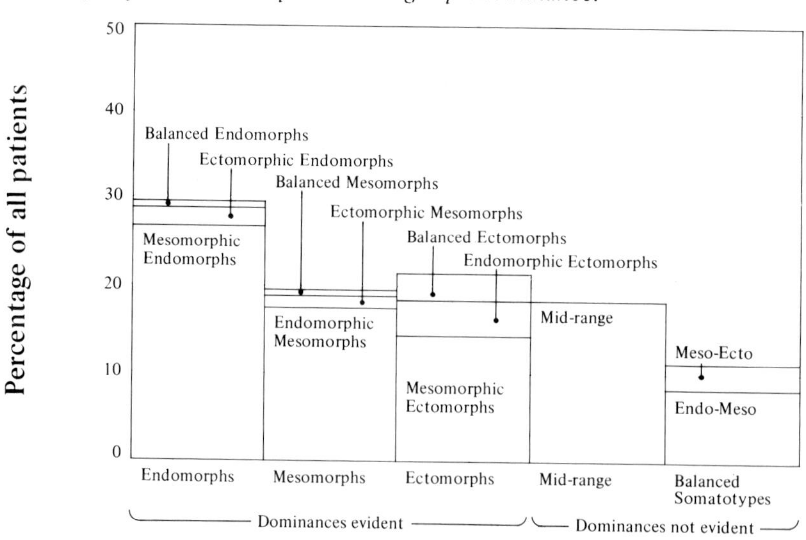

Permission to reproduce granted by Harvard University Press and M. M. Gertler, P. D. White, *Coronary Heart Disease in Young Adults* (Cambridge: Harvard University Press, 1954), p. 56. Copyright 1954 by The Commonwealth Fund.

endomorphy; the differences between the percentages showing secondary mesomorphic and ectomorphic components were statistically significant. The percentages falling into the category of endomorphy as a whole, however, showed no significant difference.

It was noted that the ectomorphs in the coronary heart disease series were all mesomorphic ectomorphs, or well-muscled, linear men.

To summarize, in comparison with the control group, the coronary heart disease group showed:

1. About the same proportion of dominant endomorphs.
2. About twice as many dominant mesomorphs.
3. Less than half as many dominant ectomorphs.
4. About the same proportion of mid-range physiques.
5. About the same proportion of two-balanced physiques.

Distribution of the coronary group

In the somatotype system, physique is represented as a three-dimensional continuum. This method, however, can be misleading since it requires a more rigid categorization than should be made. The arbitrary separation of such types as endomorphic mesomorphs, as seen in this study, creates a dichotomy not found in nature. Because of this, an alternative method devised by Sheldon was applied. The method essentially entails plotting the distribution of cases directly on the somatotype triangle. Here adjacent points are related somatotypes, whether the dominances are the same or not. As we mentioned earlier, the components are directions, and the equal-interval increments are distances along these directions. Thus, for a two-dimensional surface, the three components can be represented as three equal-length vectors, and the resultant figure is shown to be a triangle.[8] On this figure any somatotype can be plotted according to its vector position and then read.

When we plot the 97 young male patients in the coronary group, we note a clumping in the upper left sector of the triangle, an absence of peripheral positions, and a concentration in the mesomorphic sector. We see that the distribution of coronary heart disease cases clumps in the massive, "northwest" corner. (See Figure 5.3.)

In contrast, our control group of 146 males shows a more general distribution, a wider spread, and a more equitable division (though with some degree of skewing).

Table 5.9 Dominant physiques in coronary heart disease group of 97 males and unmatched control group of 146 males

	Coronary group Per cent	Control group Per cent
Endomorphs	25.7	29.9
Mesomorphs	42.2	19.8
Ectomorphs	7.3	21.1
Mid-range	17.5	18.4
Two-balanced	7.3	10.8

Permission to reproduce granted by Harvard University Press and M. M. Gertler, P. D. White, *Coronary Heart Disease in Young Adults* (Cambridge: Harvard University Press, 1954), p. 55. Copyright 1954 by The Commonwealth Fund.

Figure 5.3 Somatotype distributions of coronary heart disease group of 97 males and unmatched control group of 146 males. The patients showed a marked deficiency in ectomorphy and a deficiency in endomorphy. The physique distribution in their group was more compact.

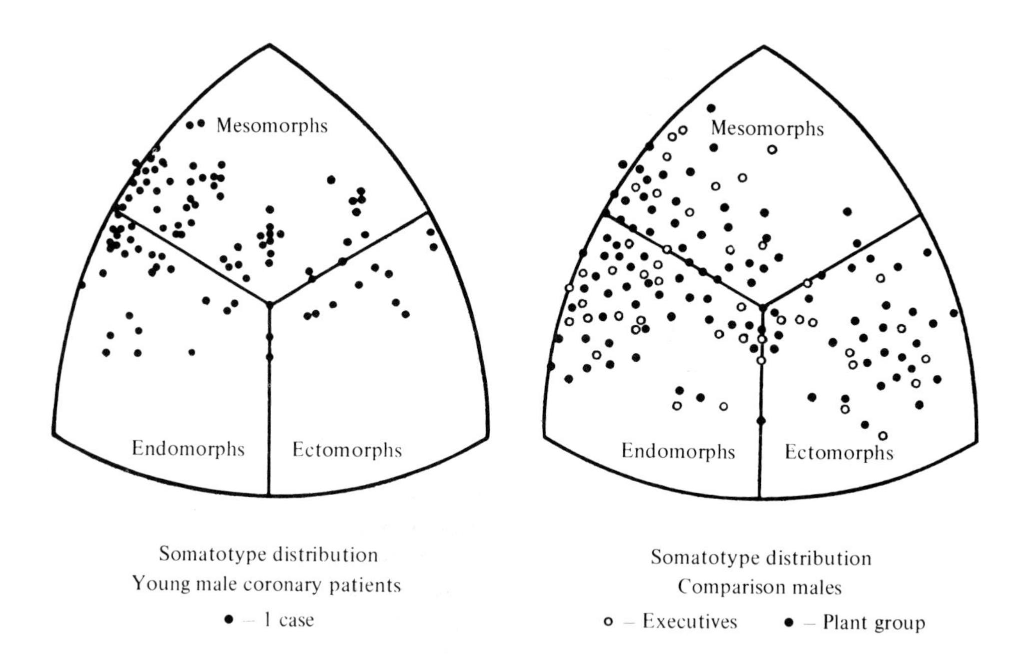

Permission to reproduce granted by Harvard University Press and M. M. Gertler, P. D. White, *Coronary Heart Disease in Young Adults* (Cambridge: Harvard University Press, 1954), p. 58. Copyright 1954 by The Commonwealth Fund.

The distribution in the lower region of the somatotype triangle is especially noteworthy; while the endomorphs and ectomorphs with low mesomorphy are well represented in the control group, the comparable area is blank for the coronary heart disease group.

Studies by Other Investigators

In the more recent literature there is a lack of agreement on which somatotype is most clearly related to heart disease. Paul's group found that there was an excess of coronary cases in the group characterized by endomorphic dominance, although it did not reach statistical significance.[9] Paul's material did not support our findings of mesomorphic dominance and endomorphic secondary dominance, though his data on somatotype is quite interesting. He observed a large proportion of mesomorphic dominance in his population, that is, 1,022/1,790 or 57 per cent. This is far greater than the normal distribution of 20 per cent for the U.S. population. Paul found only 253 patients with endomorphic dominance in his cohort of 1,790, or 14.1 per cent, whereas the normal distribution is 30 per cent for the U.S. population. The data showed 19 endomorphs with C.H.D. and 43 mesomorphs with C.H.D. Though there is a difference of opinion on which somatotype predominates among coronary patients, there is unanimity on one point: There are fewer ectomorphic dominances in the coronary heart disease group.

Working with autopsied individuals, Spain and his associates confirmed the predominance of mesomorphy in 63 per cent of their cases, with a small number of dominant endomorphs and ectomorphs, or 8 per cent, with a mixed group of 22 per cent.[10] It has been reported from Sweden that 55 post-acute coronary males were divided into two classifications: those high in cholesterol and characterized by muscle, fat, and bone, and those not exhibiting these characteristics.[11] Bjurulf found that in 110 necropsied cases there was a correlation between the degree of atherosclerosis and subcutaneous fat thickness, with bicep girth correlated for labile fat, which points to mesomorphic dominance with an endomorphic secondary dominance.[12] Spain, Nathan, and Gellis concluded from their study of 5,000 males that endomesomorphs have a threefold risk of developing C.H.D. as compared with ectomorphs.[13]

In 1969, Damon and his associates published an encyclopedic review of the role body build plays in heart disease.[14] The methodology employed by Damon for assessing body build was not the classically accepted method espoused by Sheldon and emphasized in our study. Instead, multiple regression equations were derived from the variables of height, weight, ponderal index, chest depth, upper arm circumference, triceps, subscapular skinfolds, and grip strength, which predicted somatotype within what were considered to be acceptable limits of error in various groups. The multiple coefficients of correlation between predicted and actual (that is, photographic) somatotype were significant. The regression equation was then applied to those males in the Framingham Study from whom measurements had been taken. The degree of success in predicting each somatotype was appraised by squaring the multiple correlation coefficient, which represented the per cent of variance explained by the independent variable; that is, $(0.84)^2$ = 70 per cent for endomorphy, $(0.71)^2$ = 50 per cent for mesomorphy, and $(0.91)^2$ = 83 per cent for ectomorphy.

The chief criticism of this technique lies in the fact that the coefficients of multiple correlation for the three somatotype components account for only 50-83 per cent of the total variance in predicting the actual (photographic) somatotype. The assumption that somatotype can be assessed by body measurements may be one of the reasons the Framingham body study did not completely confirm the results of this or other studies reported in the literature. The lack of confirmation of our results may also be a result of the small sample size comparable to our age group in all heart disease categories studied. Another explanation for the difference in results may lie in the difference in the body build measurements studied. The authors employed only three of the 23 indices of our original study (that is, height, weight, and chest depth) and included four measurements not studied by our group (that is, upper arm girth, triceps skinfold, subscapular skinfold, and hand grip). Gynandromorphy, also studied by Damon's group, was absent as a significant finding in both studies.

The question of whether body measurements or somatotype should be employed to assess risk of myocardial infarction naturally arises from these results. In the original linear regression formula developed by this research team, body build was responsible for 4 per cent of the contribution to risk. Damon, on the other hand, employed a discriminant function of the variables and produced a stronger relationship to C.H.D. than that of somatotype alone. Damon reported that an extended analysis was made by the Biometrics Branch of the National Heart Institute that tested this discriminant function as a single variable in conjunction with other risk factors. The results of this analysis revealed that "In general it is possible to discriminate men who will develop C.H.D. from men who will not by using body measurements alone . . . This discrimination is independent of cigarette smoking, serum cholesterol, and systolic blood pressure . . . Weight as such is not an essential discriminator."[15] The discriminant function employing body measurements in conjunction with other variables had not been used, however, to assess its singular contribution to the risk of myocardial infarction.

Although Damon's results indicated that both endomorphy and mesomorphy contributed to the nonmyocardial manifestations of early coronary heart disease, there was a failure to confirm the specific relationship of somatotype to myocardial infarction. In the age group 35-49, which was comparable to the group originally described in 1954, there appeared to be significant differences in endomorphy and ectomorphy between the various C.H.D. and non-C.H.D. categories (see Table 5.10). There was no apparent difference between the non-C.H.D. and the M.I. group for any of the somatotypes. This seems incongruous for the following reason: The category of all types of C.H.D., which included myocardial infarction and angina pectoris (generally a precursor of C.H.D.), was significantly different from the non-C.H.D. group when compared for endomorphy and ectomorphy. If this category was significant, why shouldn't the M.I. category also have been significant?

Evaluation of Weight

In the past the terms "overweight" and "obesity" were interpreted in many different ways. Because of this, the role of weight in coronary heart disease was difficult to assess. "Overweight" is, at best, a statistical concept referring to gross weight in excess of some standard selected for comparison. "Obesity," on the other hand, is a morphological concept, referring to softness, corpulence, and fatty deposits. Although it is possible to set objective standards of obesity so that individual judgments can be validated (as by the use of the constant-tension calipers by Franzen[16] or the McCloy fat calipers), ordinarily no such standards are set, and the interpretation depends to a large degree on the personal bias of the investigator, which is, in turn, a function of his experience and clientele. Despite this objection to the term, the concept of obesity has real pertinence in clinical study, for one can view directly the encompassing fatty deposits and decide whether the subject is carrying more fat than is useful. This firsthand evaluation is far superior to any table norms.

The difficulty in rating obesity and the even greater difficulty in trying to make the rating on a cadaver or from hospital records, rather than directly, have led to the practice of making determinations of overweight a measure of obesity. Overweight ratings customarily mean (a) any value above an arbitrary norm, (b) some fixed value above a norm,

*Table 5.10 The relationship of somatotype to heart disease in Framingham males aged 35-49, modified after Damon**

	Number	Mean	S.D.	p<
Endomorphy				
No C.H.D.	795	3.67	0.80	
All types				
C.H.D.	55	3.88	0.66	.03
All types				
C.H.D.–no M.I.	26	4.13	0.78	.01
M.I.	29	3.65	0.55	ns
Mesomorphy				
No C.H.D.	795	4.66	0.66	
All types				
C.H.D.	55	4.80	0.52	ns
All types				
C.H.D.–no M.I.	26	4.99	0.53	.01
M.I.	29	4.63	0.48	ns
Ectomorphy				
No C.H.D.	795	2.96	0.93	
All types				
C.H.D.	55	2.66	0.80	.01
All types				
C.H.D.–no M.I.	26	2.40	0.85	.001
M.I.	29	2.90	0.68	ns

(p values compare each group with No C.H.D.)

*A. Damon et al., "Predicting Coronary Heart Disease From Body Measurements of Framingham Males," *J. Chron. Dis.* 21: 783-785, 1969. Permission to reproduce granted by Microform International Marketing Corporation, exclusive copyright licensee of Pergamon Press Journal back files.

or (c) some fixed percentage above a norm. Furthermore, overweight must be considered in terms of the individual; it is obvious that the simple word "overweight" does not describe physique.

More recently, investigators have utilized the skinfold measurements in an effort to better distinguish obese individuals from overweight individuals. Unfortunately, there have been instances in which muscle mass or skeletal variation was not taken into consideration when body weight classifications were determined, though skinfold measurements were taken.

The original coronary study by this group did not attempt skinfold measurements, nor were these parameters measured in the follow-up study.

The relevance of skinfold measurements to body build and heart disease may be seen in the results of several investigators. Paul observed a significant difference in the mean triceps and scapular skinfold thicknesses of coronary and noncoronary groups.* Keys and his associates, in their 15-year follow-up study of a group of Minnesota

***Upper arm skinfold**–the skinfold parallel to the long axis of the right arm over the triceps area.
Infrascapular skinfold–the skinfold below the lower border of the right scapula.

Table 5.11 Comparison of coronary and control groups in 1949 and 1971 for height and weight

	Number	Height Mean ± S.D.	t	p<	Number	Weight Mean ± S.D.	t	p<
(1949)								
Controls	146	176.5 ± 6.5	5.913	.001	146	176.6 ± 24.2	2.285	.05
Coronaries	99	171.5 ± 6.3			99	169.2 ± 26.0		
(1971)								
Controls	110	177.0 ± 6.6	2.231	.05	111	182.2 ± 29.5	−0.645	ns
Coronaries	20	173.5 ± 5.8			20	177.7 ± 24.4		
(1949)								
Surviving coronaries	21	173.7 ± 6.0	1.810	ns	21	172.9 ± 23.3	0.751	ns
Expired coronaries	76	170.8 ± 6.4			76	168.1 ± 26.7		
(1949)								
Controls with C.H.D.	23	175.6 ± 6.0	2.862	.01	23	174.1 ± 26.0	0.817	ns
Coronaries	99	171.5 ± 6.3			99	169.2 ± 26.0		
(1949)								
Controls with C.H.D.	23	175.6 ± 6.0	−0.639	ns	23	174.1 ± 26.0	−0.541	ns
Controls without C.H.D.	123	176.6 ± 6.6			123	177.1 ± 23.9		
(1971)								
Controls with C.H.D.	13	175.0 ± 6.1	−1.146	ns	13	168.6 ± 25.6	−1.785	ns
Controls without C.H.D.	97	177.3 ± 6.6			98	184.0 ± 29.7		

Height determinations for 1949 and 1971 are in centimeters.

businessmen, found that a relationship exists between blood pressure and both relative weight and the sum of skinfolds.[17]

To study the problem of overweight, we followed the method of Levy et al. (1946) and computed the deviation between a norm (for height and age for each person) and actual weight.[18] This was accomplished for both the coronary heart disease group and the unmatched group of 146 controls.

The comparison between the coronary heart disease patients and the unmatched controls was also made in terms of five-year age groups—21-25, 26-30 and so on—with reference to the appropriate norms. Both the coronary and control group showed excessive weight with reference to an Army norm. The amount of excessive weight varied from age group to age group, the largest being in the 26-30-year category. However, the pattern of excess weight by age was essentially the same in the coronary group and the unmatched control group. The average deviations from the Army norms were + 19.1 pounds and + 18.5 pounds, respectively.[19]

Such criteria must be based on factors of age, sex, body build, and height. The Army standard of age, height, and weight partially fulfill these requirements; the resulting weight norms serve as a baseline with which any group may be compared. If two groups have been compared with the baseline, it is valid to compare them with each other. This was done in the present study, with the result that both the coronary and the unmatched controls represented a good cross section of the American population. The logical implication is that the entire American male population is overweight. The unsatisfactory nature of "norms" that suggest the deviation of an entire population from "normal" is evident. However, until more adequate criteria are developed, these norms serve as a valid baseline for comparison of data.

Results of the follow-up

The data on the surviving and deceased coronaries and controls revealed certain interesting trends (see Table 5.11). The original 146 controls were taller and heavier than the 100 members of the coronary group. In 1971, the surviving controls were, of course, still taller than the surviving coronaries, but there was no weight difference. In the coronary group there was also no difference in height and weight between the long- and short-term survivors. The 23 controls who subsequently developed C.H.D. were taller but not heavier than the original C.H.D. group. The control group that developed C.H.D. and those without C.H.D. did not show any difference in height and weight when compared to each other in 1949 or 1971.

The results of the follow-up reaffirm our contention that a one-to-one relationship does not exist between weight and C.H.D. The delta values of the coronary survivors revealed no changes in weight over a period of close to 25 years. The control group survivors were, on the average, 6.2 pounds heavier than they were at the start of the study. Controls who developed C.H.D. were similar to the surviving C.H.D. group in that neither showed a significant change in weight over the 25-year period the groups were followed. This is in contrast to the surviving controls without C.H.D. who gained weight to a significant degree, or 6.7 pounds. Thus, the surviving controls who did not develop C.H.D. gained weight during the course of the study without having an increased incidence of C.H.D. This becomes even more difficult to explain to those investigators

Table 5.12 Delta values of weight for coronary and control groups

	Number	Mean ± S.D.	t	p<
Coronary group	20	4.15 ± 19.87	0.934	ns
Control group	111	6.20 ± 21.37	3.057	.01
Controls without C.H.D.	98	6.77 ± 21.37	3.136	.01
Controls with C.H.D.	13	1.92 ± 21.66	0.320	ns

who believe that overweight is positively associated with C.H.D. when one considers that the controls who developed C.H.D. had no significant weight gain (see Table 5.12).

There have been many studies since 1950 that have attempted to assess the relationship of obesity to C.H.D., but there is no unanimity of opinion. The chief difficulty in these studies is not only in defining the meaning of the terms but also in ascertaining the true contribution of obesity to C.H.D. Does obesity constitute a single defined risk factor, or does it operate through other risk factors such as cholesterol, uric acid, diabetes, and hypertension? There are many studies that demonstrate that "losing weight" or restoring somatotype weight to normal will correct the other risk factors. The difficulty in evaluating obesity and/or overweight and its relationship to C.H.D. is made apparent by studying the recent literature on this subject.

The earliest Framingham Study associated only "gross" overweight or obesity with an increased rate of C.H.D.[20] However, in a later publication this concept was altered when the group reported that a weight gain after the age of 25 was strongly associated with the risk of angina pectoris and sudden death but unassociated with the development of myocardial infarction. The index of weight employed (that is, relative weight) was derived from the distribution of weight in relation to height in the total cohort.[21]

Epstein observed in his Tecumseh, Mich., study that relative weight (based on a regression of body measurements) is a definite risk factor and not merely the result of an association between high blood pressure and overweight, although it is a less potent risk factor than either blood pressure level or serum cholesterol.[22] However, Epstein cautioned in his review "to keep an open mind on the relationship between coronary disease and obesity in that an accurate analysis of the single contribution of any one variable in a disease where there are complex interrelationships is greatly dependent upon a large sample size."[23]

The Albany Study produced data suggesting that an increase in body weight of 40 per cent above the norm was associated with an increased risk of C.H.D.[24] Weight study has attempted to define overweight and/or obesity in terms of body build. Thus, a 5'10" mesomorph at 135 pounds is no more underweight than a 5'10" mesomorph is overweight at 180 pounds. The Keys Minnesota Study bears out this fact. Keys reported that men above the median weight, body fatness, and cholesterol tended to show an increased incidence of C.H.D.[25] However, when he considered relative weight as an isolated factor, it was virtually unimportant as a risk factor. Stamler et al. came to the conclusion that extreme overweight, which in reality could be interpreted as meaning overweight for one's somatotype, is associated with susceptibility to C.H.D., but that it is usually associated with C.H.D. in conjunction with other risk factors such as hypertension and diabetes mellitus. It is possible, Stamler believes, that obesity which is unassociated with hyperlipidemia, hypertension, diabetes mellitus, cigarette smoking, or other risk factors, is unrelated to proneness to coronary heart disease, except when it is extreme.[26]

Summary

Despite the evidence that obese, overweight, and heavier individuals in general did not live as long as individuals who approached normal weight, the vagueness of the terms "obese" and "overweight" was troublesome. The instrument needed for scientific accuracy came about with Sheldon's classical description of body build, which we employed in our original and follow-up studies.

There were 10 anthropometric measurements that showed significant differences between the groups (see Table 5.1). The control group, it should be noted, was slightly heavier than the coronary group (177.0 versus 170.5 pounds), and the measurements revealed that the coronary disease group had less linearity and was generally more compact, as evidenced by the ponderal indices of the group (see Table 5.3). The Sheldon description had differentiated between the body configurations of the coronary group, revealing a predominance of fat muscular persons, or endomorphic mesomorphs, while the least dominant were the slender and lean individuals, the ectomorphs. The coronary group averaged 42.2 per cent mesomorphs, compared with 19.8 per cent in the control group. On the other hand, there were 21.1 per cent ectomorphs in the control group, compared with 7.3 per cent in the coronary group.

It was of some interest to note that the surviving members of the coronary group were more linear, or ectomorphic, than the deceased coronary group (see Table 5.4). Another feature that manifested itself during the follow-up studies was the increased shoulder breadth in the survivors. This may be related to increased vital capacity because of the associated higher chest breadth resulting in a decreased chest ratio.

The original work on the somatotype associated with anthropometric measurements has been confirmed by several investigators. More interesting, however, is the observation that body build and well-chosen anthropometric measurements may be employed as a single prediction variable independent of the other risk factors.

References

1 R. E. Glendy, S. A. Levine, and P. D. White, "Coronary Disease in Youth: Comparison of 100 Patients Under 40 With 300 Persons Past 80," *JAMA* 109: 1775-1781, 1937; A. J. French and W. Dock, "Fatal Coronary Arteriosclerosis in Young Soldiers," *JAMA* 124: 1223-1237, 1944; G. A. Goldsmith and F. A. Willius, "Body Build and Heredity in Coronary Thrombosis," *Ann. Int. Med.* 10: 1181-1186, 1937; F. H. McCain, E. H. Kline, and J. S. Gilson, "A Clinical Study of 281 Autopsy Reports on Patients With Myocardial Infarction," *Am. Heart J.* 39: 263-272, 1950.

2 W. M. Yater, A. H. Traum, W. G. Brown et al., "Coronary Artery Disease in Men Eighteen to Thirty-nine Years of Age," *Am. Heart J.* 36: 334-372, 481-526, 683-722, 1948.

3 A. R. Moritz and N. Zamcheck, "Sudden and Unexpected Deaths of Young Soldiers," *Arch. Path.* 42: 459-494, 1946.

4 P. D. White, *Heart Disease* 3rd ed. (New York: Macmillan Co., 1944), p. 529; M. Newman, "Coronary Occlusion in Young Adults," *Lancet* 2: 409-411, 1946.

5 T. R. Dawber, W. B. Kannel, and G. D. Friedman, "Vital Capacity, Physical Activity and Coronary Heart Disease," in *Prevention of Ischemic Heart Disease: Principles and Practice,* W. Raab, ed. (Springfield, Ill.: Charles C. Thomas, 1966), pp. 254-265.

6 G. D. Williams, "Hereditary Aspects of Arterial Hypertension in Relation to Arteriosclerosis" in *Arteriosclerosis: a Survey of the Problem,* E. V. Cowdry, ed. (New York: Macmillan Co., 1933), pp. 537-562.

7 W. H. Sheldon, S. S. Stevens, and W. B. Tucker, *The Varieties of Human Physique* (New York: Harper Bros., 1940), p. 64.

8 Sheldon, *Varieties of Human Physique*, p. 118.

9 O. Paul, M. H. Lepper et al., "A Longitudinal Study of Coronary Heart Disease," *Circulation* 28: 20-31, 1963.

10 D. M. Spain, V. A. Bradess, and G. Huss, "Observations on Atherosclerosis of the Coronary Arteries in Males Under the Age of 46: A Necropsy Study With Special Reference to Somatotypes," *Ann. Int. Med.* 38: 254-277, 1953.

11 O. Forssman and B. Lindegard, "The Post-Coronary Patient," *J. Psychosomatic Res.* 3: 89-169, 1958.

12 R. Bjurulf, "Atherosclerosis and Body Build," *Acta Med. Scand. Suppl.* 166, 1959.

13 D. M. Spain, D. J. Nathan, and M. Gellis, "Weight, Body Type and the Prevalence of Coronary Atherosclerotic Heart Disease in Males," *Am. J. Med. Sci.* 245: 63-68, 1963.

14 A. Damon, S. Damon, H. C. Harpending, and W. B. Kannel, "Predicting Coronary Heart Disease From Body Measurements of Framingham Males," *J. Chron. Dis.* 21: 781-802, 1969.

15 Damon, "Predicting Coronary Heart Disease," p. 802.

16 R. Franzen, "Physical Measures of Growth and Nutrition," in *School Health Research Monographs*, No. 2 (New York: Am. Child Health Assoc., 1929), pp. 1-138.

17 A. Keys, H. L. Taylor et al., "Coronary Heart Disease Among Minnesota Business and Professional Men Followed Fifteen Years," *Circulation* 28: 381-395, 1963.

18 R. L. Levy, P. D. White, W. P. Stroud, and C. C. Hillman, "Overweight: Its Prognostic Significance," *JAMA* 131: 951-953, 1946.

19 S. M. Garn, M. M. Gertler, S. A. Levine, and P. D. White, "Body Weight Versus Weight Standards in Coronary Artery Disease and a Healthy Group," *Ann. Int. Med.* 34: 1416-1420, 1951.

20 T. R. Dawber, F. E. Moore, and G. V. Mann, "Coronary Heart Disease in the Framingham Study," *Amer. J. Publ. Hlth.* 47(4): 4-24, 1957.

21 W. B. Kannel, E. J. LeBauer, T. R. Dawber, and P. M. McNamara, "Relation of Body Weight to Development of Coronary Heart Disease," *Circulation* 35: 734-743, 1967.

22 F. H. Epstein, L. D. Ostrander et al., "Epidemiologic Studies of Cardiovascular Disease in a Total Community–Tecumseh, Michigan," *Ann. Int. Med.* 62: 1170-1187, 1965.

23 F. H. Epstein, "The Epidemiology of Coronary Heart Disease: A Review," *J. Chron. Dis.* 18: 735-774, 1965.

24 J. T. Doyle, A. S. Heslin, H. D. Hilleboe, and P. F. Formel, "Early Diagnosis of Ischemic Heart Disease," *New Eng. J. Med.* 261: 1096-1101, 1959.

25 Keys, Taylor et al., "Coronary Heart Disease," pp. 381-395.

26 J. Stamler, D. M. Berkson, H. A. Lindberg et al., "Coronary Risk Factors," *Med. Clin. No. Am.* 50: 229-253, 1966.

VI Biochemical Findings: The Interrelations of Serum Lipids

Historical Background

Historians claim that around 1769 Pouletier de la Salle first called attention to a substance in gallstones that was soluble in alcohol and formed crystals upon evaporation.[1] Chevreul, in 1824, repeated de la Salle's experiments and named the substance "cholesterol" (chole=bile, steros=solid).[2] Denis (1830) is credited with having been the first to report that blood serum contains cholesterol.[3]

Possibly the earliest association between cholesterol and atherosclerosis was made in 1847 when Vogel observed that cholesterol was present in atherosclerotic lesions.[4] Windaus analyzed various diseased aortae in 1910 and reported six times as much cholesterol and 20 times as many cholesterol esters in atherosclerotic aortae as had been observed in normal aortae.[5] Schoenheimer (1928, 1934) and others extended these observations and concluded, after performing chemical analyses of many aortae, that the proportion of lipids in the aorta increased with age and atherosclerosis.[6]

From these observations, investigators, both clinical and experimental, began studying the interdependence of the level of serum cholesterol and the degree of atherosclerosis. Experimentalists, led by Anitschkow and Chalatow (1913), produced atherosclerosis in rabbits by feeding them large quantities of cholesterol.[7] Clinicians attempted to learn whether the incidence of atherosclerosis in people with hypercholesterolemia was higher than in the normal population. Thus, individuals with hereditary hypercholesterolemia,[8] nephrosis,[9] hyperthyroidism,[10] xanthomatosis,[11] and diabetes mellitus[12] were studied to ascertain the incidence of atherosclerosis.

Both methods of approach have had their opponents and proponents. Duff (1935) objected to Anitschkow's conclusions on the grounds that cholesterol, an animal sterol, might have an effect as an unnatural factor in a herbivorous diet of human beings, which commonly includes animal sterols.[13] Leary (1949), on the other hand, came to the same conclusions as Anitschkow after repeating Anitschkow's experiments and studying human autopsy material with a polarizing microscope.[14]

The measurement of cholesterol in the blood serum has assumed greater importance since vast epidemiological studies were first begun. Since 1950, the study of the intermediate metabolism of cholesterol synthesis has been clarified to a large extent, albeit not completely. Concomitant with the elucidation of cholesterol synthesis has been the advent of hypercholesterolemic drugs that have been employed to lower serum cholesterol and, hence, theoretically remove an important risk factor in atherosclerogenesis of the coronary arteries.

Cholesterol Synthesis

Although the chemical formula of cholesterol, $C_{27}H_{46}O$, was suggested by Reinitzer in 1888, its molecular structure has been a subject of controversy for many years.[15] Through the efforts of many investigators, however, the structure has been accepted, subject to change, as a phenanthrene-cyclopentane or "cholane" form of sterol ring. The pathway of steroid synthesis is similar for most steroids up to a certain point: The cyclopentenoperhydrophenanthrene ring is formed, then the side chains, double bonds, oxygen, and hydroxy groups are added to make the specific steroid. Thus the unsaturated alcohol, cholesterol, is closely related to bile acids, cortisone, estrone, and testosterone.

Bloch confirmed that cholesterol was derived from acetate by showing that ^{14}C-labeled acetate was found in squalene as well as cholesterol, both in vivo and in vitro from liver and liver slices.[16] This confirmed Robinson's earlier work, which suggested that squalene was an intermediate in cholesterol biosynthesis.[17] The same investigator demonstrated not only that both carbons from acetate were involved in this synthesis but that the entire molecule could be derived from acetate. Other groups soon entered into the study of uncovering the basic synthetic pathways. Wright and Folkers made an important discovery by determining the mode of synthesis of mevalonic acid from acetate.[18]

Lipid synthesis and atherosclerosis

The advances in biochemical techniques have been extended to the study of atherosclerogenesis. Electron microscopy, fluorescent and ferritin-conjugated antibody studies, radioautography, tissue culture, and histoenzymology have all been utilized in an attempt to solve the problem of atherosclerogenesis. Such methodology has virtually supplanted the purely descriptive and analytical techniques of the past half-century. The rate of incorporation of ^{14}C-labeled cholesterol in the intima and media of various arteries, it has been found, gives a clue about the rate of endogenous cholesterol synthesis in the arteries. The greatest source of arterial cholesterol in contrast to phospholipids appears to be a local synthesis.[19] The studies employing acetate-2-^{14}C incorporation into individual lipids and protein indicate that (a) the lipids are better synthesized in the fatty streaks than in the intima, (b) phospholipids are the major lipids synthesized in both the intima and the fatty streaks, and (c) intimal synthesis contributes to the marked accumulation of lipids in the fatty streaks.[20]

The questions that remain are: (a) What is the detailed composition of the lipids and other materials in the various arterial layers? (b) What is the source of these materials—are they exogenous or endogenous? (c) What is the secondary effect of these accumulated materials on the arterial composition itself? The literature indicates that intimal tissue accumulates lipids of all types during a lifetime.[21] The distribution is both perifibrous and in droplet form throughout the intima. The main component of these lipids is cholesterol linoleate in the form of Sf 0-12 lipoproteins in the perifibrous tissue and cholesterol oleate in the fat-filled droplets. During the abnormal or disease state, the lipid content is charged both quantitatively and qualitatively with new lipids, such as sphingomyelin, lecithin, free cholesterol, and cholesterol oleate in the fat-filled cells. In the fibrous distribution of the diseased aortae, the accumulation is mainly sphingomyelin and cholesterol linoleate. Thus, the essential difference is one of quantity and not quality.

It is generally agreed that lipids can enter through the intima. Free cholesterol penetrates the arterial wall with much greater ease than esterified cholesterol or triglycerides. Since cholesterol, phospholipids, triglycerides, and free fatty acids were usually found together in lipoproteins, it was natural to try to determine whether lipoproteins entered the artery. It was observed by conjugating fluorescein and lipoproteins that both low and very low density lipoprotein antibodies appeared in the smooth muscle cells of the intima. There was not, however, a definite relationship between the degree of lipoprotein deposit or lipid deposit in the arteries and the composition of the serum lipids themselves.

What is the source of these materials? The answer is not final, but there is evidence that phospholipids, as well as cholesterol and cholesterol esters, may be synthesized in the aorta. Furthermore, there is a question as to whether a hyperlipemic diet influences the rate of protein synthesis, accumulation, and catabolic processes within the arterial smooth muscle cells, or if it induces cellular damages that proceed to atherosclerosis. Again, the evidence is not conclusive at this time.

In keeping with observations in humans, recent animal experiments have described inconsistencies in the theory that cholesterol per se is causally related to atherosclerogenesis.[22] Studies of this type are divided into natural sequences, such as the relationship of dietary lipids to plasma lipids and the formation of lipid deposits within the arterial wall. The animal experiments show a latitude of species difference. In rabbit studies, cholesterol is added to the normal rabbit's low-fat diet. This maneuver results in hyperlipemia, which is not only the result of hypercholesterolemia but also hyperphospholipidemia and hypertriglyceridemia. Rabbits fed diets high in carbohydrates, in the form of glucose and starch, also display hyperlipemia.[23]

Although hyperlipemia may be produced in other animals such as swine,[24] rats,[25] and rhesus monkeys,[26] the techniques of feeding, alteration of the thyroid with thiouracil, pancreatectomy, and cholic acid supplements all demonstrate that hyperlipemia is not a matter of a simple relationship between dietary intake and serum alteration. These animal experiments parallel observations in men and women in other parts of the world. The levels of serum cholesterol and their relationship to atheropoiesis in various countries leave doubt as to the true significance of this variable outside the United States.

There appears to be some relationship between diet and the level of serum cholesterol, but this remains open to further study. Many factors, including intake, excretion, absorption, hormonal influences, degradation, and species difference, are intertwined in this heterogeneous problem. The question also arises as to what relationship, if any, exists between hyperlipemia of various types and degrees, and lipid deposition within the arteries. The answer is not readily available because there appear to be inconsistencies in the observations.

The evidence from the use of ^{3}H-labeled thymidine strongly suggests that hyperlipemic serum produces a stimulatory effect on smooth muscle cells.[27] Studies employing ^{32}P- and ^{14}C-labeled acetate suggest that phosphatidylcholine is also synthesized at a more rapid rate in arteries containing hyperlipemic serum. The best available evidence suggests a change in basic cellular metabolism in aortas during the aging and atherosclerotic processes. There seems to be unanimity of opinion that as atheropoiesis proceeds, the combined ratio of free cholesterol and cholesterol esters to the phospholipid moiety is increased greatly. There has been evidence of an uncoupling of oxidative phosphorylation in aortic mitochondria of hyperlipemic rabbits. Free fatty acids and triglycerides remain essentially unchanged.

There is another aspect of atheropoiesis that is important to consider: Arterial tissue has a unique property that is otherwise observed only in malignant tumors, the retina, and muscle, and which produces large amounts of lactic acid in the presence of oxygen in contrast to the rate of anaerobic glycolysis.[28] Thus the Pasteur effect (the regulation of lactic acid production by glycolysis), which parallels the Kreb's cycle oxidation rate, is lost and excessive lactic acid is produced. Such evidence supports the observations that arterial walls contain large amounts of glycogen that may serve as an energy source during low oxygen tension. This could be an important metabolic clue in understanding how such cofactors as TPN (triphosphopyridine nucleotide), DPN (diphosphopyridine nucleotide), NAD (nicotinamide-adenine dinucleotide), and NADP (nicotinamide-adenine dinucleotide phosphate), along with its reduced form, NADPH (produced from aerobic glycolysis of the arterial tissue), serve in the synthesis of the lipids and cholesterol within the arterial wall. Theoretically, with greater deposit of lipids there is a decreased oxygen supply and greater dependence on aerobic glycolysis with resultant lipid and cholesterol synthesis. One could speculate that exercise reverses this process by increasing oxygenation and reducing the inhibition of the Pasteur effect.

In addition to the theories portraying atherosclerosis as a purely lipid disease, there is one school of thought that relates atherosclerogenesis to a blood clotting defect. This theory dates back to Rokitansky et al.[29] and has had strong proponents in Mallory[30] and Clark et al.,[31] who extended Rokitansky's view with more refined studies and observations. It remained, however, for Duguid et al. to study this problem in depth at a time when the concepts of blood coagulation were being advanced at a rapid rate.[32] Duguid suggested that the fibrous thickenings observed on the intima were a result of surface deposition from blood platelets and other materials. Duguid reasoned that if the fibrous thickenings were due to a local phenomenon, the arteries would lose their elasticity due to replacement and loss of elastic tissue, and dilate in accordance with the systolic expansion normally observed. Thus Duguid's theory and observations, although not totally accepted, have credibility and merit. It would appear that several processes are working together to produce the lesions observed: lipid deposition and local synthesis; fibrous deposition; degeneration and calcification, coupled with endothelialization; and, finally, thrombus formation.

Still another viewpoint merits mentioning at this time. The structure of the coronary arteries with their bifurcations, branchings, bends, and narrowings are subjected to continuous pulsatile stresses from the systolic and diastolic pressure changes. These hemodynamic forces, coupled with the histological structure and anatomical variations described above, produce pressure and flow phenomena that may be described in actual physical terms, as in Poiseuille's, Bernoulli's, or Reynold's equations.[33] Several investigators have suggested that the shear and drag at these vulnerable points make these sites particularly prone to atherosclerogenesis.

Thus, despite the many detailed and elegant reports in the literature that employ tracers and the electron microscope, the limits on the physical resolution powers available today have made it difficult to demonstrate conclusively the mechanisms of hyperlipemic serum or a causal relationship between it and other changes that may be associated with atherosclerosis.

Lipid Values

In addition to the determination of the absolute level of serum total cholesterol in the coronary heart disease group and a matched control group of healthy men, the question of the influence of such factors as age, weight, body build, and diet on the level of serum total cholesterol was considered and interpreted in the present study with particular reference to the range of the normal level and its etiologic relation to coronary heart disease. Since cholesterol was shown to be only one of the variables involved in the etiology of C.H.D., other lipids, such as phospholipids, were also determined in both groups. The interrelations of the various lipids were also considered because of the current viewpoint that the colloidal state of all substances within the serum is more important than any one individual substance.

The Bloor methods[34] for determining cholesterol esters were employed throughout the original study. Serum phospholipids were determined by the Fiske and Subbarow technique.[35] In our determinations, lecithin was expressed as 25 times the lipid phosphorus value (the amount of organic phosphorus in the total lipids of the serum).

In 1949, the average levels of cholesterol esters and total cholesterol were significantly greater in the coronary heart disease group than in the matched control group. The mean serum levels of phospholipids and free cholesterol were also higher in the disease group than in the control group, although not to a significant degree. The distribution of the two groups for serum cholesterol was studied and considerable overlap was found, that is, 22 matched controls exceeded the mean value of the coronary group (286 mg per cent) and, conversely, 27 coronary subjects fell below the mean of the matched control group (241 mg per cent). See Figure 6.1.

In the follow-up study, cholesterol was determined by the Abell (et al.) technique,[36] lipid phosphorus by the Fiske and Subbarow method,[37] and triglycerides by the Van Handel and Zilversmit technique.[38]

The serum cholesterol values were examined in the coronary and control groups in diverse combinations (see Table 6.1). In 1949, we found a significant difference between the control and coronary groups in serum cholesterol ($p<.001$). This difference was also evident in 1971 when the surviving groups were examined.

In comparing the cholesterol values for the 23 controls who subsequently developed C.H.D. with the original coronary group, it was found that in 1949 there was a significant difference between these two groups ($p<.001$). It would be reasonable to assume, in the light of present-day knowledge, that serum cholesterol would have been of great predictive value in the 23 controls who developed C.H.D. On close examination, however, this was not found to be the case. In 1971, when these two groups were compared, no difference in serum cholesterol was observed. Essentially, the surviving C.H.D. group and the surviving controls with C.H.D. were similar in this respect.

If cholesterol were causally related to C.H.D. or even strongly associated with C.H.D., one would expect the 1949 cholesterol values of the surviving controls who

Table 6.1 Significant differences in serum cholesterol levels between coronary and control groups at initial and follow-up examinations

	1949 Number	1949 Mean ± S.D.	1949 t	1949 p<	1971 Number	1971 Mean ± S.D.	1971 t	1971 p<
All controls	146	225 ± 43	8.44	.001	114	228 ± 39	3.66	.001
All coronaries	98	288 ± 75			20	263 ± 47		
Controls with C.H.D.	23	233 ± 33	1.00	ns	14	241 ± 47	1.33	ns
Controls without C.H.D.	123	223 ± 43			100	226 ± 37		
Controls without C.H.D.	123	223 ± 43	−8.06	.001	100	226 ± 37	−3.91	.001
All coronaries	98	288 ± 75			20	263 ± 47		
Controls with C.H.D.	23	233 ± 33	−3.45	.001	14	241 ± 47	−1.38	ns
All coronaries	98	288 ± 75			20	263 ± 47		
Deceased controls with C.H.D.	8	239 ± 31	−0.65	ns				
Surviving coronaries	21	248 ± 57						
Controls with C.H.D.	23	233 ± 33	−1.09	ns				
Surviving coronaries	21	248 ± 57						
Deceased coronaries	74	295 ± 67	−2.95	.01				
Surviving coronaries	21	248 ± 57						

Figure 6.1 Level of serum total cholesterol in coronary heart disease group, unmatched control group, and matched control group. The distributions within the histogram are not discontinuous; however, there were more individuals with coronary heart disease whose cholesterol exceeded 300 mg. %, while there were more in the control groups whose serum cholesterol was less than 210 mg. %.

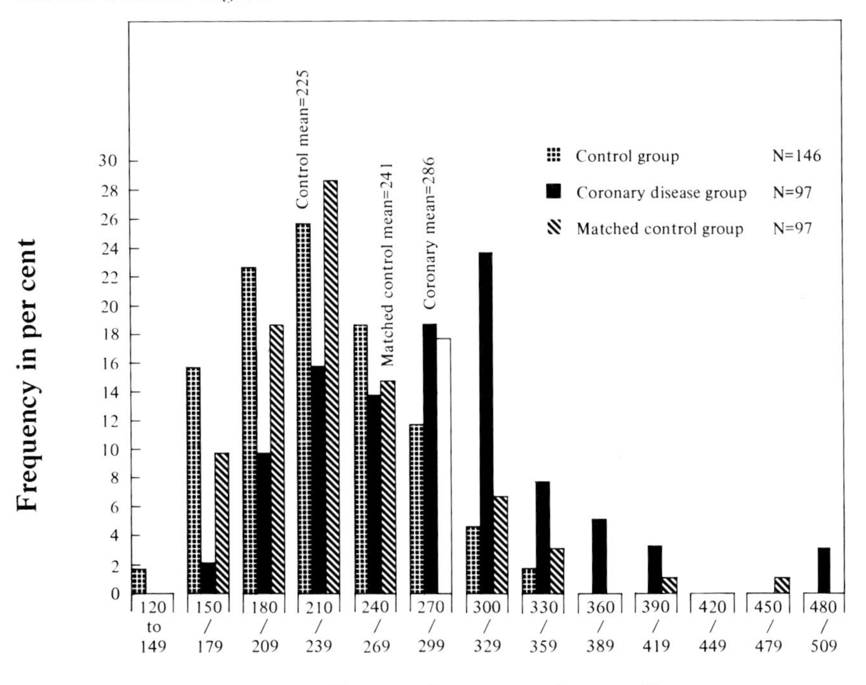

developed C.H.D. to be lower than those of the deceased controls who developed C.H.D. This was found to be the case, although the difference was not statistically significant.

In 1949, the 123 controls who did not develop C.H.D. and the original C.H.D. subjects had serum cholesterol values of 223 mg per cent and 288 mg per cent, respectively. The difference between these two groups was statistically significant ($p < .001$). These findings were similar to those found in the entire control group when compared to the original coronary group in 1949. The same findings were observed when the surviving members of these two groups were compared in 1971.

When the 23 controls who developed C.H.D. were compared to the 21 surviving coronaries for 1949 serum cholesterol values, no significant differences were found. These two groups resembled each other. Similar results were observed when the 1971 values were compared, as reported earlier.

The controls who did not develop C.H.D. and the controls who did develop C.H.D. had serum cholesterol values in 1949 of 223 mg per cent and 233 mg per cent, respectively. One might have expected a higher serum cholesterol in the controls with C.H.D., which was found, but it was not statistically significant. The same results were observed when the two groups were compared in 1971.

The most dramatic expression of the value of serum cholesterol as a predictor of survival in the coronary group was derived from the 1949 data. The average serum cholesterol in 1949 of those members of the original coronary group who have since expired was 295 mg per cent. This value was significantly higher than that of the surviving members of the coronary group (248 mg per cent). These data offer some insight into the predictive value of cholesterol in survival in a disease group.

It should be recalled that the histograms of serum cholesterol levels in the coronary and control groups overlapped a great deal. Accordingly, those members whose serum cholesterol levels were 0.5 to 1.0 standard deviations below the mean values of the C.H.D. group had better survival records.

Our observations that early mortality in the C.H.D. group appeared to be related to levels of serum cholesterol were in contrast to the observations of Frank, who found no relationship between levels of hypercholesterolemia and second heart attacks.[39] The early reports from the Coronary Drug Project could not support Frank's viewpoint but stated that more information would be required, although preliminary data permitted the conclusion that there was a 20-30 per cent increase in mortality with high cholesterol levels. However, the recent data from the Coronary Drug Project indicate that there was no difference in mortality in men whose serum cholesterol was lowered by clofibrate or niacin when compared to a placebo group.[40] Thus, men whose serum cholesterol attained values of less than 250 mg per cent had death rates of 20.4, 21.5, and 19.7 in the clofibrate, niacin, and placebo groups, respectively. Similarly, men in the clofibrate, niacin, and placebo groups whose serum cholesterol attained values of more than 250 mg per cent had a mortality rate of 19.6, 20.8, and 22.3 per cent, respectively.

Data from the Scottish[41] and Newcastle[42] studies showed a significantly lower death rate among angina patients in the clofibrate-treated groups than in the placebo groups. This is in contrast to the results of the Coronary Drug Project. Both studies agreed, however, that there was a lack of correlation between their results, the initial serum cholesterol levels, and the degree of response to clofibrate treatment. The studies showed that the beneficial effects of clofibrate may be of even greater importance to the prognosis of coronary heart disease survival in terms of decreased fibrinogen levels and increased fibrinolysis,[43] and reduction in abnormal platelet stickiness.[44] Thus, the lipid-lowering effect of clofibrate on cholesterol, free fatty acids, and triglycerides may actually influence the clotting mechanisms, whose changes may be masked by the more easily measured lipid effects. The relationship of lipids to the clotting mechanism is discussed in Chapter VIII.

The three studies indicate that once serum cholesterol is elevated and the disease process has continued for a period of time, reversal of serum cholesterol levels will not necessarily affect the mortality rate, regardless of the method employed in achieving this effect. It appears in the case of clofibrate that the favorable results may be related not only to cholesterol lowering but also to other effects that clofibrate purportedly possesses. Accordingly, the evidence from these studies permits one to conclude that perhaps there are additional factors that should be included in an intervention study to prevent coronary events. This view has been espoused by the authors for more than two decades.

From the data on our series of coronary and control subjects, it seems that the initial serum cholesterol level is a good predictor of survival in C.H.D. patients who have survived a myocardial infarction. Serum cholesterol proved to be of limited value as a risk factor in distinguishing those controls who would subsequently develop C.H.D., and it was only a limited indicator of survival probabilities in this same group.

Delta values of serum cholesterol

It is interesting to follow the changes in serum cholesterol within both the initial coronary group and the control group over the past 25 years. No statistically significant changes in serum cholesterol were noted in either the surviving coronary or control groups (with or without C.H.D.). However, the surviving coronary group did show the greatest increase, or 16.1 mg per cent (see Table 6.2). The original value of 248 mg per cent for the surviving C.H.D. group was low when compared to the deceased C.H.D. group mean of 295±67 (see Table 6.1). The controls who subsequently developed C.H.D. did show a greater increase in cholesterol over the past 25 years than did the controls who did not develop C.H.D., although not to a statistically significant degree.

Age and Serum Cholesterol

Today the predominant evidence indicates that there is a rise in serum lipids in males, whether one refers to cholesterol, cholesterol esters, phospholipids, Sf molecules, or beta lipoproteins. The descriptions of the cumulative curves usually emphasize a rise in serum lipids during the preteen and the teen-age years, which continues until the 4th or 5th decade. At that time, the serum lipids begin to decline gradually until the 7th, 8th, and 9th decades. The same general trend applies to women, where the actual lipid levels are somewhat more elevated in later age.

Many papers have been written on this subject since the first edition of this monograph appeared. For the most part they have confirmed the findings presented therein, while others have extended the original observations in both younger and older age groups. Table 6.3 is a summary of the major reports concerned with age and serum cholesterol.

Figure 6.2 is a composite of cholesterol levels for the American population, but it does not reflect international levels.

Table 6.4 summarizes the findings in the C.H.D. group, the matched control group,

Table 6.2 Delta cholesterol of surviving coronary and control groups in mg. %

	Number	Mean ± S.D.	t	p<
Coronary group	20	16.10 ± 59.09	1.2185	ns
Control group	114	3.12 ± 45.64	0.7297	ns
Controls with C.H.D.	14	9.79 ± 35.79	1.0234	ns
Controls without C.H.D.	100	2.19 ± 46.94	0.4665	ns

Table 6.3 Mean serum cholesterol levels by sex and age for specified populations

Sex and age	Total U.S. HES 1960-62	Framingham 1958-60	Tecumseh, Mich. 1959-60	Evans Co., Ga. 1960-62
Men				
25-34	207	–	205	203
35-44	228	233	221	220
45-54	231	237	233	223
55-64	234	235	229	226
65-74	230	–	224	221
75-79	225	–	–	–
Women				
25-34	198	–	196	199
35-44	214	217	212	221
45-54	234	246	230	237
55-64	265	262	251	259
65-74	267	–	256	260
75-79	245	–	–	–

Permission to reproduce granted by the National Center for Health Statistics, U.S. Department of Health, Education, and Welfare, Vital Health Statistics, *Serum Cholesterol Levels of Adults– United States 1960-62,* Series 11, No. 22, p. 7.

Figure 6.2 Composite of mean cholesterol levels of major U.S. heart disease study groups for different age groups

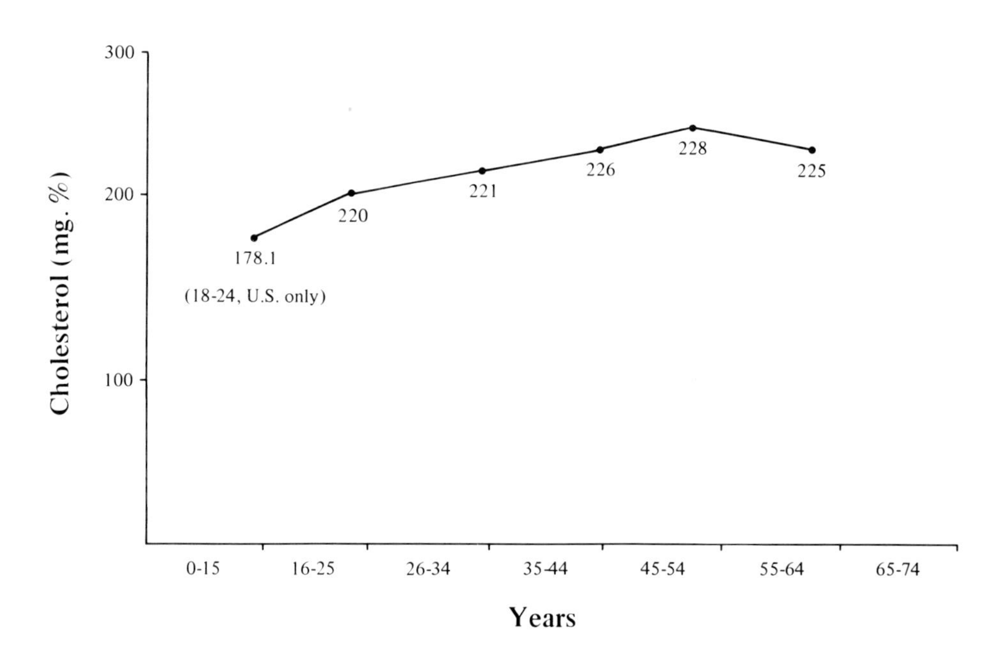

Table 6.4 Serum total cholesterol in coronary heart disease, matched control, and control groups–1949 determination

Age	Controls		C.H.D.		Matched controls	
	Number	Mean ± S.E.	Number	Mean ± S.E.	Number	Mean ± S.E.
20-29	20	195 ± 9.2	7	245 ± 27	7	230 ± 12
30-39	74	224 ± 4.8	53	286 ± 9	53	227 ± 5
40-49	46	236 ± 6.0	35	301 ± 11	32	246 ± 8
50-59	6	254 ± 13.5	2	259	2	242

Table 6.5 Coefficients of correlation (r) with serum cholesterol (1), serum phospholipids (2), and age (3) in healthy adult men and in men with coronary artery disease*

	Normals		Coronary artery disease	
	Number	r	Number	r
r_{12}†	146	.66 ± .05	61	.51 ± .09
r_{13}	146	.30 ± .08	95	.16 ± .10
r_{23}	146	.42 ± .07	61	.20 ± .12

*Phospholipids are expressed as lecithin, which is considered to be 25 times the blood lipid phosphorus level.

†r_{12} means that coefficient of correlation is between serum cholesterol and serum phospholipids.

Only 61 phospholipids out of 62 were taken simultaneously with serum cholesterol.

Permission to reproduce granted by The American Heart Association, Inc. and M. M. Gertler et al. *Circulation* II(4): 517-522, 1950.

and the control group with respect to age and serum cholesterol for 1949 cholesterol determinations. Note that the matched control group resembles the C.H.D. group more than does the control group. This is emphasized by the observation that significant differences occurred between the controls and the C.H.D. group and not between the matched controls and the C.H.D. group.

The rise in serum cholesterol with age must be considered in relation to the rise in serum phospholipids as well. Tables 6.5 and 6.6 illustrate this point.[45]

It is apparent from Table 6.5 that the phospholipids are highly correlated with cholesterol and show even higher correlations with age than does cholesterol in both the healthy and the coronary disease groups. Since all three variables were intercorrelated, it was decided to employ the technique of partial correlation, which would theoretically determine the primary correlations of any pair of variables with the third held constant. The significance of this correlation will be discussed later. These correlations are tabulated in Table 6.6.

It is apparent from Table 6.6 that (a) in both health and coronary artery disease, the cholesterol-phospholipid correlation is higher independent of age; (b) the correlation between cholesterol and age disappears when the influence of phospholipids is removed;

Table 6.6 Partial correlations among cholesterol (1), phospholipids (2), and age (3) in the serum of healthy adult men and men with coronary artery disease

	Healthy controls		Coronary disease group	
	Number	Partial correlation	Number	Partial correlation
$r_{12.3}$*	146	.62 ± .05	61	.50 ± .10
$r_{13.2}$	146	.05 ± .08	95	.07 ± .10
$r_{23.1}$	146	.32 ± .07	61	.14 ± .13

*$r_{12.3}$ means that the partial correlation is between cholesterol and phospholipids with age kept constant.

Permission to reproduce granted by The American Heart Association, Inc. and M. M. Gertler et al. *Circulation* II(4): 517-522, 1950.

and (c) the phospholipids tend to remain correlated with age in the healthy group, but they may not keep pace with age in coronary artery disease.

The difference between the two partial coefficients of correlation (.32±.07 in health and 0.14±.13 in coronary artery disease) does not reach significance ($p=0.20$), probably because of the small size of the coronary sample, but there is other evidence that the phospholipids play an altered role in coronary artery disease.*

The role of phospholipids and other lipids in atherosclerogenesis has been alluded to in the earlier sections of this chapter. A very neglected aspect is the relationship of serum phospholipids and other lipids to the clotting mechanism, which also plays a major role in the atherosclerotic process.

Race and Serum Cholesterol–International Studies

There are unconfirmed claims that atherosclerosis is practically unknown among such peoples as the Chinese, Eskimos, and Okinawans, whose diet is purported to contain very little cholesterol and whose serum total cholesterol is said to be lower than that of the American population. However, a survey made by the Coronary Research Laboratory did not substantiate any relation between ingested cholesterol and the level of serum total cholesterol (see Chapter VIII).

It is apparent that coronary heart disease occurred in our study with greater frequency in individuals who might be classified as the mid-Mediterranean ethnic group. We did not investigate this question completely, but we did analyze the findings in two groups of individuals–Jews and Italians. Since individuals of Jewish origin were numerous in the series, the levels of serum total cholesterol were determined both for them and for the non-Jewish population of the C.H.D. group and the matched control group.

In the coronary heart disease group there was a small and not statistically significant difference in the level of serum total cholesterol between the Jews and non-Jews. In the matched control group the difference was somewhat larger but in the opposite

*Permission to reproduce granted by The American Heart Association, Inc. and M. M. Gertler, S. M. Garn, P. D. White, "Age, Serum Cholesterol, and Coronary Artery Disease," *Circulation* II(4): 517-522, 1950.

Table 6.7 Mean cholesterol of healthy populations age 40-59 years in various countries (modified after Keys)

	Number	Mean cholesterol (mg. %)
Dalmatia (Croatia)	672	186
Slavonia (Yugoslavia)	699	198
West Finland	817	253
East Finland	860	265
United States	–	238
Crevalcore (Italy)	993	200
Montegiorgia (Italy)	719	200
Zutphen (Netherlands)	–	230
Crete (Greek Island)	686	202
Corfu (Greek Island)	529	198
Tanushimaru (Japan)	509	170
Ushibuka (Japan)	504	140

Source: A. Keys, "Coronary Heart Disease in Seven Countries," *Circulation* 41(4) Suppl. 1: 1-211, 1970.

direction; it was also not statistically significant. Although the cholesterol levels in the Jews of the coronary heart disease group exceeded those of the matched control Jews, the difference was not statistically significant; but between the non-Jewish coronary and control groups there was a significant difference.

The six Italians in the coronary heart disease group were compared in a similar way with the six Italians in the matched control group. The average serum total cholesterol for those with coronary heart disease was 278.15 mg per cent, while for the six in the matched control group it was 253.0 mg per cent. In a group so small this is not a significant difference.

There is no doubt that data in the United States indicate that the level of serum cholesterol is associated with atheropoiesis. Data from several sources in the United States may be refined to the degree where an accurate estimate may be given concerning the probability of C.H.D. events as related both to time and level of cholesterol.

The application and transference of the data accumulated in the United States to other populations has failed to be as accurate or confirmatory of the statistical applications as they are utilized in this country. Since one of the chief parameters in the statistical evaluation is serum cholesterol, the reasons are apparent why the calculations cannot be simply transposed from the United States to the cohorts of other populations, since their serum cholesterol levels are much lower (see Table 6.7).

The examination of data from various sections of north, mid, and south India, the U.S.A., and Japan indicates that serum cholesterol rises in men between the ages of 21 and 51. The absolute levels are also lowest in the Asian countries and highest in the U.S.A. (see Tables 6.8 and 6.9).

Cholesterol studies in other countries show that serum cholesterol levels are higher in individuals with C.H.D. than in controls. However, there are many countries where the levels of serum cholesterol in C.H.D. are lower or equal to the normal values in the United States, such as India, Pakistan, and Yugoslavia. Such data from international sources have a common denominator—the presence of C.H.D.—but the difference in the levels of

Table 6.8 Mean normal values of serum cholesterol according to different authors

	Age 21-30 Mean ± S.D.	Age 31-40 Mean ± S.D.	Age 41-50 Mean ± S.D.	51 and above Mean ± S.D.
Mathur et al. (1959) India	159 ± 25	170 ± 42.6	178 ± 42.4	188 ± 17.4
Padmavati et al. (1959) India	164 ± 25	174 ± 40	172 ± 22.5	150 ± 30
Srikantia et al. (1961) South India	161 ± 9.6	173 ± 5.3	175 ± 5.1	174 ± 16.0

Source: K. S. Mathur, N. P. Wahi, K. K. Malhotra, R. D. Sharma, and S. K. Srivastava, "Dietary Fats, Serum Cholesterol and Serum Lipid Phosphorus in Different Socioeconomic Groups in Upper Pradesh," *J. Ind. Med. Assoc.* 33: 303, 1959; S. Padmavati, S. Gupta, and G. V. Pantula, "Dietary Fat, Serum Cholesterol Levels and the Incidence of Atherosclerosis in Delhi," *Circulation* 19: 849, 1959; S. G. Srikantia, S. N. Jagannathan, and S. Gopalan, "Serum Cholesterol and Blood Pressure Levels in Some South Indian Population Groups," *Ind. J. Med. Res.* 49: 99, 1961.

Table 6.9 Mean serum cholesterol of U.S. and Japanese adults (1960-62, 1958-60) according to age and sex

	United States mean cholesterol	Japanese mean cholesterol		United States mean cholesterol	Japanese mean cholesterol
Men			Women		
30-39	219	150	30-39	208	152
40-49	231	157	40-49	224	161
50-59	231	157	50-59	258	177
60-69	233	160	60-69	265	179

Permission to reproduce granted by the National Center for Health Statistics, U.S. Department of Health, Education, and Welfare, Vital Health Statistics, *Serum Cholesterol Levels of Adults–United States 1960-1962,* Series 11, No. 22, p. 7.

Table 6.10 Mean serum cholesterol in C.H.D. patients and controls in various countries

	Mean age	Mean ± S.D.	p<
India			
Coronary group	40	199 ± 49	.001
Control group	40	176 ± 43	
Pakistan			
Coronary group	37	214.5	.01
Control group	36	184.2	
Yugoslavia			
Coronary group	54	236.5 ± 48	.001
Control group	44	210.9 ± 32	

Source: I. J. Pinto, F. Colaco, "Risk Factors in Ischemic Heart Disease in Lower Socio-Economic Class in Bombay, India," in *The First International Biennial Conference on Cardiac Rehabilitation* (Tisak, Rijecka Tiskara, Rijeka, 1970), p. 119; M. Beg, M. Zafar, M. Raza, G. A. Hashmi et al. "Risk Factors of Vascular Disease in Pakistan," in *The First International Biennial Conference on Cardiac Rehabilitation* (Tisak, Rijecka Tiskara, Rijeka, 1970), p. 145; R. Dimnik, "Analogous Metabolic Studies on Coronary Patients and Healthy Subjects," in *The First International Biennial Conference on Cardiac Rehabilitation* (Tisak, Rijecka Tiskara, Rijeka, 1970), p. 151.

serum cholesterol suggests that this may not be the universal common factor in C.H.D., a view held with great tenacity until recently (see Table 6.10).

Physique and Serum Cholesterol

Determination of the differences between the levels of the various lipids for the various dominant physiques is imperative, not only to establish the meaning of normal lipid levels, but also to determine the difference, if any, that exists between (a) the physiques in any one group and (b) similar physiques in any two groups. Since physical constitution is predetermined to a large degree, it is reasonable to suppose, without postulating any degree of association or causal relation, that the chemical attributes such as serum cholesterol and serum uric acid may also be genetically determined. Hence, an attempt to associate physique with serum lipids has certain theoretical justification.

This has been done, in the past, in studies that correlated the levels with various physiques.[46] The reliability of these studies is necessarily limited by their haphazard system of physique classification and their ill-defined terminology (see Chapter V). To avoid as much as possible the limitations described above, without placing undue stress on ratios or index scales of build, the Sheldonian system of body build rating was selected for use in this work.[47]

In Table 6.11 the values of the four lipids—free cholesterol, cholesterol esters, total cholesterol, and phospholipids—are listed under physical groups, which have been classified into primary dominances for the coronary and unmatched control groups. Comparisons were also made between the means of the four major physical categories, both within and between the unmatched control group and the coronary heart disease group (see Figure 6.3).

In evaluating the relation of morphological characteristics to the level of serum total cholesterol, it should be kept in mind that in an average population the levels in endomorphs, mesomorphs, and mid-range individuals exceed the levels in ectomorphs. At the age of 35, the mean levels of serum total cholesterol for the ectomorphs and the other groups combined would be 207 mg per cent and 224 mg per cent, respectively. Abnormal levels would assume the values of 207±74 mg per cent and 224±84 mg per cent, while high but not abnormal levels would assume values of 207±37 mg per cent and 224±41 mg per cent, respectively.

The further interrelation of age and morphological characteristics with the level of serum total cholesterol is now apparent. While these figures do not include enough individuals for a complete age-morphological survey, it is reasonable to suggest that an ectomorph at any age would possess, on the average, a lower level of serum cholesterol than would individuals with other physiques (see Figure 6.2).

Lipoproteins

During the early 1950s, Gofman et al. studied serum lipoprotein structure in the ultracentrifuge. Gofman devised an analytic flotation method based on Svedberg's work in Sweden. This work gave a strong impetus to the biochemical investigations of C.H.D. Gofman reported his characterization of lipoproteins as Sf units of various degrees of

Table 6.11 Serum lipids, by physiques, in coronary heart disease group of 97 males and unmatched control group of 146 males (Mean ± S.E., mg. %)*

Physique	Number of cases	Free cholesterol	Number of cases	Cholesterol esters	Number of cases	Total cholesterol	Number of cases	Phospholipids†
Endomorphs								
coronary	24	113.51 ± 9.4	24	176.0 ± 11.7	25	286.8 ± 12.9	19	310.6 ± 11.7
control	51	101.51 ± 4.1	51	133.1 ± 4.8	51	234.6 ± 6.6	51	311.3 ± 5.8
difference		ns		‡		‡		ns
Mesomorphs								
coronary	43	110.2 ± 5.1	43	184.2 ± 7.0	43	294.4 ± 9.3	27	319.5 ± 10.5
control	34	104.3 ± 4.4	34	119.0 ± 4.1	34	223.3 ± 6.2	34	300.3 ± 6.0
difference		ns		‡		‡		ns
Ectomorphs								
coronary	9	100.4 ± 11.5	9	164.1 ± 16.4	9	264.6 ± 19.8	5	328.0 ± 12.0
control	34	96.8 ± 4.6	34	111.0 ± 4.4	34	207.8 ± 6.0	34	281.2 ± 6.4
difference		ns		§		‡		‡
Mid-range								
coronary	18	111.6 ± 19.0	18	165.8 ± 15.2	20	279.1 ± 16.3	11	314.0 ± 19.0
control	27	94.0 ± 5.6	27	133.4 ± 6.3	27	227.4 ± 8.2	27	298.3 ± 7.5
difference		ns		§		‡		ns
Total								
coronary	94	110.4 ± 3.9	94	176.7 ± 5.5	97	286.5 ± 6.6	62	316.4 ± 6.7
control	146	99.7 ± 2.3	146	124.7 ± 2.6	146	224.4 ± 3.5	146	299.3 ± 3.3
difference		§		‡		‡		§

*In 3 cases, free cholesterol and cholesterol esters were not determined.
In 35 cases, lipid phosphorus (phospholipid) determinations were not made.
†Phospholipids are expressed as 25 times the lipid phosphorus.
‡Significant at the 1% level.
§Significant at the 5% level.
ns–Not significant.

Permission to reproduce granted by Harvard University Press and M. M. Gertler, P. D. White, *Coronary Heart Disease in Young Adults* (Cambridge: Harvard University Press, 1954), p. 109.

Figure 6.3 Serum total cholesterol levels in coronary heart disease group and unmatched control group. Within the coronary group, mesomorphs had a higher level of serum total cholesterol than endomorphs or ectomorphs. Within the control group, endomorphs had a higher level of serum total cholesterol than mesomorphs or ectomorphs. A comparison of the coronary with the control group shows higher levels in the coronary group for all physiques, the largest difference occurring in the category of mesomorphy.

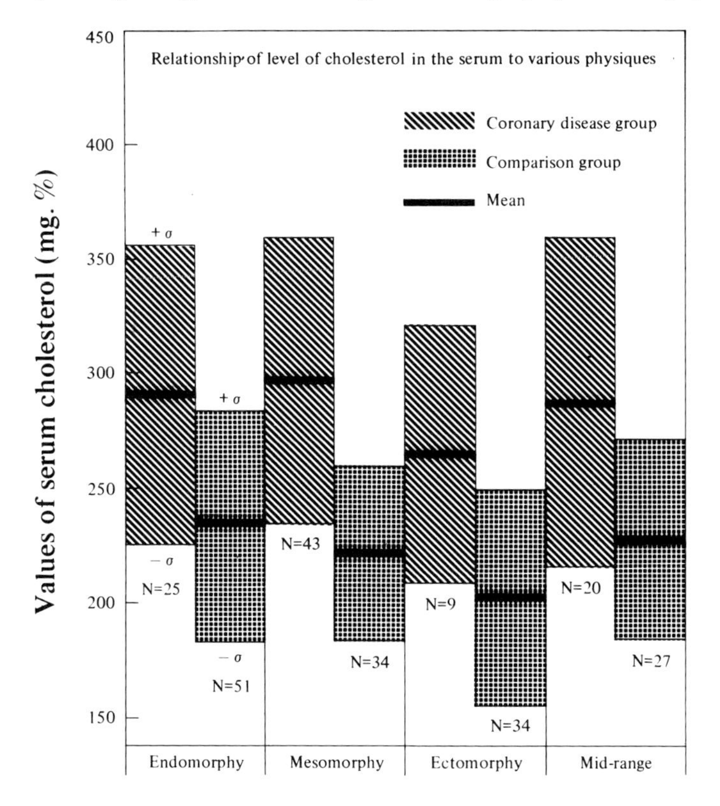

Permission to reproduce granted by Harvard University Press and M. M. Gertler, P. D. White, *Coronary Heart Disease in Young Adults* (Cambridge: Harvard University Press, 1954), p. 110. Copyright 1954 by The Commonwealth Fund.

migration from the zero point. Essentially, in the study of C.H.D. there appeared to be two groups of special interest: low density lipoproteins (1.05 gm/mm or less) and high density lipoproteins, where the densities are above 1.5 gm/mm. There appeared to be a strong correlation between Sf 12-20 lipoprotein class and C.H.D., although a contribution from Sf 20-100 and Sf 100-400 classes was involved. These classes were analyzed and found to have varying amounts of cholesterol, phospholipids, and neutral fats.[48]

Hyperlipoproteinemia consists basically of alpha and beta lipoproteins. Alpha lipoproteins are composed of about 50 per cent protein and 50 per cent lipid. The lipid

Table 6.12 Cholesterol and protein concentrations in lipoprotein patterns (modified after Lees)

Lipoprotein classification	L.D.L. protein (mg. %)	L.D.L. cholesterol (mg. %)	C/P ratio
Normal	83	140	1.7
I	40	28	0.7
II	129	236	1.8
III	71	154	2.2
IV	103	135	1.3
V	75	78	1.0

Source: R. S. Lees, "Immunoassay of Plasma Low-Density Lipoproteins," *Science* 169: 493-495, 1970.

composition is 44 per cent phospholipids, 28 per cent cholesterol esters, 6 per cent unesterified cholesterol, 17 per cent glycerides, and about 6 per cent or less unesterified fatty acids. Beta lipoproteins are composed of approximately 25 per cent protein and 75 per cent lipid. The lipid composition is 46 per cent cholesterol esters, 14 per cent unesterified cholesterol, 25 per cent phospholipids, 14 per cent glycerides, and about 1 per cent or less unesterified fatty acids.

Gofman's work was not extended to clinical levels for many reasons, one of which was the technical difficulty that would have evolved from mass assays. Lees, however, extended Gofman's work by developing an immunoassay for determining the concentration of the protein moiety of the low density lipoproteins in human plasma.[49] This method was developed because there appeared to be theoretical reasons for suspecting that, even though low density lipoproteins (L.D.L.) were associated with C.H.D., there were quantitative differences within the L.D.L. insofar as the cholesterol and protein concentrations were concerned. Lees found that the protein moiety varied according to the lipoprotein patterns as observed in Table 6.12, which is modified from his data.

It is interesting to note that the highest values are found in type II and type IV. Lees concluded on the basis of his studies that since many individuals with type IV lipoprotein pattern and C.H.D. have normal L.D.L. cholesterol, L.D.L. protein could be a far better predictor than either serum cholesterol or L.D.L. cholesterol concentrations.

Levy and Fredrickson modified Gofman's assay method and extended his studies by applying a simpler paper electrophoretic method to the study of plasma lipoproteins.[50] Supplementing this with actual analyses of cholesterol and triglycerides, they devised a system that was more accurate in typing than either method alone. The description and management of the lipoprotein classifications are listed in Table 6.13.

The lipoprotein patterns were not being done at the time of the original study. In the follow-up study, however, this was possible. The following patterns were found in the control and coronary groups (see Table 6.14):

The lipoprotein classification in the follow-up studies appears to demonstrate a greater percentage of type II abnormalities in both the surviving C.H.D. patients and the surviving controls with C.H.D., the percentages being 21 and 21.4, respectively, as opposed to 7.1 per cent in the surviving controls ($p<.01$). It is interesting to note that in a different population studied at the same clinic, the predominant type for C.H.D. and

Table 6.13 Description and management of lipoprotein classifications

Class	Plasma	Cholesterol	Triglycerides	Flotation class abnormalities	Dietary management
I (very rare)	creamy	normal or elevated	markedly elevated	Sf 100-400↑	Restrict fat to 25 gm/day, supplement medium-chain-length triglycerides
II (common)	clear	elevated	IIa–normal IIb–elevated	Sf 0-12↑↑↑ 20-100↑	Low cholesterol (<300 mg/day), substitute polyunsaturated fats for saturated
III (relatively common)	clear cloudy milky	elevated	usually elevated	Sf 0-12↓ 12-100↑↑	Reduce to ideal body weight, low cholesterol (<300 mg/day), balanced diet (40% calories fat, 40% carbohydrates)
IV (common)	clear cloudy milky	normal or elevated	elevated	Sf 0-20 normal or 20-400↑↑↑	Reduce to ideal body weight, substitute polyunsaturates, moderate carbohydrate intake
V (uncommon)	creamy	elevated	elevated to markedly elevated	Sf 20-400↑	Reduce to ideal body weight, increase protein intake, reduce fats to less than 70 mg/day, restrict carbohydrates

Permission to reproduce granted by Flint Laboratories, Division of Travenol Laboratories, Inc., Morton Grove, Ill. 60053, "Primary Hyperlipoproteinemias: A Correlation of Electrophoretic Pattern, Chemical Findings, Dietary and Drug Management."

Table 6.14 Predominant lipoprotein patterns in control and coronary groups

Group	Number	Type I	Type II	Type III	Type IV	Normal
Controls without C.H.D.	99	0	7 (7.1%)	3 (3%)	21 (21.2%)	68 (68.7%)
Controls with C.H.D.	14	0	3 (21.4%)	0	1 (7.1%)	10 (71.4%)
Coronary group	19	0	4 (21%)	1 (5.3%)	3 (15.8%)	11 (57.9%)

Table 6.15 Lipoprotein distribution of a C.H.D., ITCVD, and control group

Group	Number	Type II	Type IV	Normal
C.H.D. group	45	2 (4.5%)	29 (63.4%)	14 (31%)
ITCVD group	36	2 (5.5%)	22 (6 1.0%)	12 (33%)
Control group	91	2 (2.3%)	26 (28.6%)	63 (69%)

Table 6.16 Mean phospholipids of coronary and control groups in 1949 and 1971

	1949				1971			
	Number	Mean ± S.D.	t	p<	Number	Mean ± S.D.	t	p<
Deceased coronaries	49	12.89 ± 2.1	2.25	.05				
Surviving coronaries	16	11.55 ± 2.0						
Coronaries	65	12.54 ± 2.1		ns	20	11.17 ± 1.7	2.58	.01
Controls	46	12.03 ± 1.7			113	10.09 ± 1.7		
Controls without C.H.D.	23	12.15 ± 1.4		ns	99	10.05 ± 1.8		ns
Controls with C.H.D.	23	12.01 ± 1.7			14	10.36 ± 1.5		

ischemic thrombotic cerebrovascular disease (ITCVD) was type IV.[51] (See Table 6.15.) The reasons for these differences are not entirely clear. They may be the results of the more recent diets favoring less fat in which carbohydrates are consumed in greater quantities. Similar lipoprotein distributions in accordance with this latter study have been reported by Zelis and his co-workers.[52]

Phospholipids

Phospholipids as a group are not only an integral part of the lipoproteins but are also found in the lipid deposits within the arteries. Their synthesis, which is much better understood today than it was in 1950, is a dynamic process that is highly interrelated with both lipid and carbohydrate metabolism as well as protein metabolism via the amino acids ethanolamine, choline, and serine, to mention the most important ones. In addition to being present in lipoproteins and the arterial wall, phospholipids form a large portion (63 per cent) of thromboplastin, which plays an important role in blood coagulation.

Essentially, phospholipids are composed of a nucleus of L α glycerol, which is derived from the Embden-Meyerhof, or anaerobic, phase of glucose metabolism. It is this which constitutes their relationship with carbohydrate metabolism.

1) glucose $\xrightarrow[mg]{ATP}$ glucose-6-phosphate +ADP

2) glucose-6-phosphate is eventually metabolized to

3) glycerol phosphate ⇅

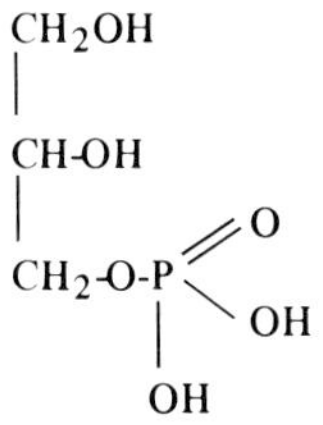

$$\begin{array}{l} CH_2OH \\ | \\ CH\text{-}OH \\ | \\ CH_2\text{-}O\text{-}P(=O)(OH) \\ \quad\quad\;\; | \\ \quad\quad\; OH \end{array}$$

4) phosphatidic acid

$$\begin{array}{l} CH_2\text{-}O\text{-}R^1 \\ | \\ CH\text{-}O\text{-}R^2 \\ | \\ CH_2\text{-}O\text{-}P(=O)(OH) \\ \quad\quad\;\; | \\ \quad\quad\; OH \end{array}$$

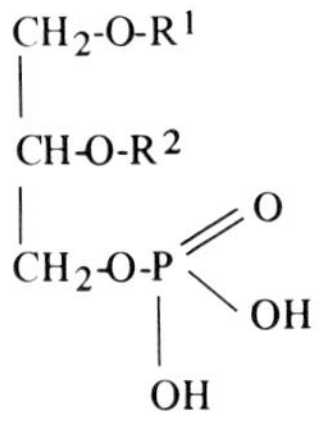

(R^1 and R^2 represent fatty acids of various lengths and saturation)

The glycerol phosphate on its 1 and 2 positions may be esterified with fatty acids of various lengths and saturation to become phosphatidic acids. This step relates the phospholipids to lipid metabolism.

The step in synthesis from phosphatidic acid to phosphatidylcholine (lecithin), phosphatidylethanolamine (cephalin), and phosphatidylserine relates the compound phospholipids to proteins. Hence, the phospholipids as compounds are interrelated with carbohydrate (glycerol), fats (fatty acids in the α and β positions), and, finally, proteins through the attachment of the amino acid position 3 to phosphate. The intermediate metabolic pathways involve cytidine diphosphate choline (ethanolamine) in a manner similar to the involvement of uridine diphosphate in carbohydrate metabolism.[53]

The phospholipids are highly active and participate in many biological oxidations. They have been considered clot-promoting substances since 1883.[54]

The results of the follow-up examination revealed a significantly higher mean phospholipid level in the 49 deceased C.H.D. patients than in the 16 surviving patients. The surviving coronary group also revealed a significantly higher phospholipid level than the surviving control group in 1971. There were no differences between those controls with and those without C.H.D. in either 1949 or 1971 (see Table 6.16).

The delta values (the change between 1949 and 1971) did reveal certain interesting

Table 6.17 Delta phospholipids of control and coronary groups

Group	Number	Mean	t	p<
Surviving C.H.D. group	15	–0.33	–0.743	ns
Surviving control group	113	–1.86	–9.936	.001
Surviving controls without C.H.D.	99	–1.95	–9.328	.001
Surviving controls with C.H.D.	14	–1.24	–4.783	.001

Table 6.18 Mean triglyceride levels in control and coronary groups in 1971

Group	Number	Mean ± S.D.
Coronary group	19	167.9 ± 94.8
Control group	112	142.2 ± 84.4
Controls without C.H.D.	98	142.7 ± 87.2
Controls with C.H.D.	14	139.1 ± 62.8

Table 6.19 Coefficient correlations in 1949 between cholesterol and selected variables in coronary and control groups

Variable	Coronary group Number	r	Control group Number	r
Height	98	–0.1849	146	–0.1395
Weight	98	–0.0950	146	0.0737
Ponderal index	98	–0.0066	146	–0.1818
Phospholipids	66	0.5118*	146	0.6597*
BUN	84	0.1244	145	0.0173
Uric acid	94	–0.0604	146	0.1232

*Significant correlation p<.001

Table 6.20 Coefficient correlations in 1971 between cholesterol and selected variables in coronary and control groups

Variable	Coronary group Number	r	Control group Number	r
Height	20	–0.2447	110	–0.0553
Weight	20	–0.0285	111	–0.0808
Ponderal index	20	–0.2028	110	–0.1433
Phospholipids	20	0.8180***	113	0.7549***
BUN	20	0.3642	112	0.1260
Uric acid	19	0.1107	114	0.1895*
Triglycerides	19	0.4431(*)	112	0.3058**

(*)Significant correlation p<.10
* Significant correlation p<.05
** Significant correlation p<.01
*** Significant correlation p<.001

trends. The C.H.D. survivors showed an insignificant drop in phospholipids, whereas there were significant decreases in phospholipids in the surviving controls both with and without C.H.D. (see Table 6.17).

In summary, the changes observed in the phospholipid levels were not indicative of a major or minor trend that would be considered helpful in assessing the present status of coronary heart disease.

Triglycerides

Studies made on the surviving coronary and control groups in 1971 and on controls with and without C.H.D. did not reveal any significant differences between the groups in triglyceride levels. The highest values did occur in the C.H.D. group (167.9 mg per cent). These observations confirm those of Albrink and colleagues, who found that triglyceride elevations were associated more with ischemic cerebrovascular disease than heart disease.[55] (See Table 6.18.)

Coefficient Correlations

The coefficient correlations between serum total cholesterol and other parameters are summarized in Tables 6.19 and 6.20. The 1949 data revealed only two statistically significant correlations: a positive correlation with phospholipids in the C.H.D. group (r=0.51) and the control group (r=0.66). In the linear regression analysis based on the 1949 data, phospholipids are protective against C.H.D.—a point that is borne out in these observations of a higher correlation group. The difference is not seen as dramatically in the 1971 data, where the level of significance in the C.H.D. and control groups is virtually the same although more significant than in 1949 (r=0.82 and 0.75, respectively). This is emphasized in an earlier publication where biserial coefficient correlations revealed that in C.H.D. the rise in serum phospholipids with cholesterol failed to parallel the rise that was observed in the control patients.[56]

Methods of Lowering Cholesterol

There is no one and only acceptable way to lower serum cholesterol. But in addition to determining the level of serum cholesterol, the lipoprotein classification should be made available, since this information may be helpful in determining what method to employ for lowering serum cholesterol.

Dietary

There is strong evidence to support a change in diet as a means of lowering cholesterol. Weight reduction does not succeed in all cases, but it may in individuals whose excessive calories are converted into excess adipose tissue, triglycerides, and cholesterol, among other substances. Weight reduction should not be carried on below the ideal accepted weight for an individual's somatotype. In some instances, this has opened the way for other disease entities to manifest themselves. Often, merely lowering the weight does not lower the serum cholesterol. One may then resort to (a) decreasing the total fat intake and (b) increasing the unsaturated fat/saturated fat ratio.

An abundance of literature indicates that dietary saturated fatty acids increase the serum cholesterol, whereas polyunsaturated fatty acids reduce the level of serum cholesterol. These observations have altered the prevailing concept relating the amount of fat intake to the level of serum cholesterol. The newer concept has been changed to include not only the amount of fat in the diet but also the type of fat ingested. Formerly, it was thought that populations that consumed only 15 per cent of their total calories in fats fared better with respect to atherosclerosis than did those populations consuming 40 per cent of their total calories in fats. However, the important effect of polyunsaturated fats was not considered in this evidence.[57]

There are a few basic facts concerning fats and cholesterol that are noteworthy. Fats with less than 12 carbon atoms usually do not affect serum lipid levels.[58] Three fatty acids, namely lauric (C_{12}), myristic (C_{14}), and palmitic (C_{16}) have profound effects on raising the serum cholesterol.[59] The polyunsaturated acids (those with two or more double bonds, such as linoleic acid) are effective as hypocholesterolemic agents. One should recognize that saturated fatty acids raise the level of serum cholesterol twice as much as the equivalent amount of polyunsaturated fatty acids lower serum cholesterol.

There is still much disagreement about the role of dietary fats in atheropoiesis.[60] However, in a statement made by the Inter-Society Commission for Heart Disease Resources, the following recommendations regarding substantial reduction of dietary saturated fats were made: "The ideal quantity of fat needed in the diet is not known, but moderation in intake is considered desirable, i.e. less than 35 per cent of total calories from all fats. Intake of less than 10 per cent of total calories from saturated fats is of critical importance for attainment of optimal serum cholesterol levels for most people. Unsaturated fats may be used in moderation to replace a portion of the saturated fats, i.e. 10 per cent of calories from mono- and up to 10 per cent from polyunsaturated fats. With proper control of saturated fat, cholesterol, and calorie intake, as recommended above, ingestion of large amounts of polyunsaturated fats–i.e., 10 per cent or more of total calories–is generally not necessary for control of serum lipid levels . . . The Commission therefore recommends that the food industry be encouraged by the medical profession and the Government and supported by the general public to make available leaner meats and processed meats, dairy products, frozen desserts and baked goods reduced in saturated fats, cholesterol and calories, and visible fats and oils (margarines, shortenings, mayonnaise, salad dressings, oils) of low saturated fat and cholesterol content."*

Such food items as skim milk, nonfat cottage cheese, safflower and corn oil, and soft safflower margarine come under these categories. The diet for an individual with type II hyperlipoproteinemia would be geared toward providing a high polyunsaturated fat ratio and restricting the cholesterol intake to less than 300 milligrams per day. A daily food plan would include one pint or more of skim milk, cooked poultry, fish, or lean trimmed meat, five servings of vegetables or fruit, seven or more servings of whole grain

*Permission to quote granted by The American Heart Association, Inc., "Report of Inter-Society Commission for Heart Disease Resources," *Circulation* 42:84, 1970.

or enriched bread or cereal, one or more servings of potato, rice, etc., allowed fat, and allowed dessert.

The diet for an individual with type IV hyperlipoproteinemia would be geared toward attaining and maintaining "ideal" body weight and controlling carbohydrate intake as well as moderately restricting cholesterol and modifying fat intake.

Hypocholesterolemic agents

The newer knowledge of cholesterol synthesis has produced many new drugs that inhibit cholesterol synthesis at certain levels of its intermediate metabolism. Some of these have produced toxic symptoms, and their use has been discontinued. The three general categories of these agents are:

a) substances that interfere with cholesterol absorption:
- sitosterols (suspension)
- cholestyramine
- colestipol

b) a substance that interferes with cholesterol synthesis:
- clofibrate

c) substances that aid in cholesterol catabolism:
- niacin
- sodium dextrothyroxine

a) The sitosterols are chemically similar to cholesterol, except for an ethyl group in position 24. The most important isomer from a human viewpoint is beta sitosterol, which is virtually not absorbed, and prevents both exogenous and endogenous cholesterol from being absorbed in the intestine as well. The mechanism for this action is thought to be mixed crystal formation and increased esterification of cholesterol.[61]

Cholestyramine is a basic anion exchange resin with a unique affinity for bile acids. Cholestyramine is a polymer containing quaternary ammonium groups attached to a styrene-2 per cent divinylbenzene skeleton. The chloride anion is attached to each quaternary group and may be displaced by bile acids, since bile acids have a higher affinity for the resin than does chloride.[62]

Colestipol is a high-molecular-weight, insoluble copolymer of tetraethylenepentamine and epichlorohydrin. It is able to bind acids in vitro of 1 m.Eq. cholic acid/gm.

In preliminary trials colestipol lowered serum cholesterol and had very little effect on serum triglycerides. At concentrations of 0.5-5 per cent, the drug inhibited cholesterol-induced hypercholesterolemia in cockerels after four days. When colestipol was studied in type II hyperlipoproteinemic males, serum cholesterol was 20 per cent below levels in placebo-treated males. No untoward hematologic, hepatic, or renal damage has been reported as a result of colestipol.[63]

b) Clofibrate lowers serum cholesterol and serum triglyceride levels. In addition to this effect on blood lipids, it also has an observable effect on blood coagulation mechanisms, such as normalizing the platelet adhesiveness.

Clofibrate's mode of action has not been completely established. It is known that clofibrate causes a redistribution of several plasma-protein-bound compounds such as androgens, thyroxine, pyridoxal phosphate, and tryptophan in the liver. During treatment with clofibrate, there is an inordinate rise in NAD, NADP, and their reduced forms, while several NAD-dependent enzyme systems are unaffected. This raises two interesting questions. Inasmuch as niacin (or nicotinic acid, a cogener of NAD) also has been known to lower serum cholesterol, is the basis for lowering cholesterol secondary to NAD or NAD-dependent enzyme systems? And, are NAD and NADP involved in cholesterol synthesis?

There are other mechanisms postulated for the mode of action of clofibrate. These include a decrease in the rate of free fatty acid mobilization; blocked synthesis of cholesterol between acetate and mevalonic acid, and perhaps between mevalonic acid and cholesterol; an increase in the rate of hepatic cholesterol oxidation; a decrease in the hepatic release of lipoproteins; and an increase in the peripheral uptake of lipoproteins.[64]

c) Niacin (nicotinic acid) aids in cholesterol catabolism. There are many theories concerning the action of niacin, not one of which is entirely supportable by experimental evidence. There is speculation concerning the production of oxycholesterol,[65] heparin-like substances,[66] increased body metabolism,[67] removal of methyl group,[68] and decreased endogenous cholesterol.[69] The evidence for the action of niacin as a hypocholesterolemic agent appears to suggest more strongly a decreased cholesterol synthesis; that is, an inhibition of the process by which ^{14}C-labeled acetate is converted to cholesterol in man.[70] Niacin also reduces triglycerides by its hepatic action and its reduction of free fatty acid flow to the liver.

Sodium dextrothyroxine. The thyroid gland has been implicated with good evidence in fat and lipid metabolism. Patients with hypothyroidism tend to have higher levels of cholesterol as well as other lipids, whereas the opposite is true for individuals with hyperthyroidism.[71] The most apparent conclusion to be drawn from these facts is that L-thyroxine or its equivalent should be administered to lower serum lipids and cholesterol in an effort to reduce the risk rate of C.H.D. However, the side effects of L-thyroxine and its equivalents in producing hyperthyroidism are sufficient to discourage this form of treatment. The search for a derivative of L-thyroxine that would maintain the lipid- and cholesterol-lowering properties without having the side effects of hyperthyroidism yielded D-thyroxine. D-thyroxine is a definite cholesterol-lowering agent whose action increases the rate of degradation and oxidation of cholesterol. The effect is chiefly on cholesterol; the observations on tripalmitin, phospholipids, and triglycerides, in general, did not reveal any statistically significant alteration in the serum lipids.

Recently, however, there has been an increase in the reports of side effects—angina pectoris and deaths. Therefore, the use of D-thyroxine has been contraindicated, especially in ischemic heart disease.

Miscellaneous compounds
–nonabsorption compounds
–neomycin

There are other interesting compounds thus far not generally employed for lowering serum cholesterol. These nonabsorption compounds include (a) a hydrophilic colloid derived from the blond psyllium seed,[72] (b) Dextran and cellulose anion exchangers, which are similar to cholestyramine in action,[73] (c) DEAE-Sephadex, which achieves results similar to cholestyramine and Dextran,[74] and (d) lignin, which binds bile acids with great affinity and thus also produces results similar to Dextran.[75]

Table 6.21 Change in cholesterol biosynthesis, fecal steroid excretion, and isotopic cholesterol turnover rate after partial ileal bypass (modified after Moore et al.)

	Number of patients	Prior to surgery*	After surgery*
Synthesis	15	622	2,753
Fecal steroid excretion	3	785	2,955
Isotopic cholesterol turnover	7	930	2,804

*All values are in mg/day.

Source: R. B. Moore, I. D. Frantz Jr., R. L. Varco, and H. Buchwald, "Cholesterol Dynamics After Partial Ileal Bypass," in *Atherosclerosis: Proceedings of the Second International Symposium on Atherosclerosis* (New York: Springer-Verlag, 1970), pp. 295-300.

Table 6.22 Percentage decrease in serum cholesterol after partial ileal bypass (modified after Buchwald)

	Baseline	3 months	1 year	3 years	5 years
Number of patients	98	90	71	35	13
Mean cholesterol (mg. %)	358.5	215.7	217.9	214.2	204.2
Per cent lowered	0	40	39	40	43

Source: H. Buchwald, R. B. Moore, R. L. Varco, "Surgical Treatment of Hyperlipidemia," *Circulation* 49 (5) Suppl. 1:1-23, 1974.

It was reported by Samuel and Steiner that 1-2 grams daily of neomycin reduced serum cholesterol 10-36 per cent.[76] The mechanism was thought to be secondary to a change in intestinal flora, which would cause oxidation of sterols, reduce fat, and reduce sterol absorption.[77] There were observations on the reduction of the cholesterol pool, while there was no demonstrable effect on the decay curve.

Ileal bypass

Ileal bypass, introduced by Buchwald, Moore et al., as a way of reducing hypercholesterolemia, has sound experimental evidence to support it.[78] (See Table 6.21.)

The evidence demonstrates an increased conversion of cholesterol to bile acids and a diminished cholesterol absorption. The increased compensatory cholesterol synthesis is sufficient to maintain equilibrium with the loss described. Data that are specific on the effects of this procedure on serum cholesterol are summarized in Table 6.22, modified after Buchwald.

Exercise

Experiments by Kobernick et al. demonstrate that serum cholesterol may be lowered by prolonged treadmill running by rabbits.[79] Other more recent publications emphasize the importance of exercise not only as a form of calorie utilization but also as a factor worth employing in the prevention of ischemic heart disease. The value of a prescribed exercise program is currently being investigated by a national cooperative program sponsored by the Social and Rehabilitation Services Division of the Department of Health, Education, and Welfare. The hypotheses upon which this is based are the following:

a) Exercise is a calorie utilizer.
b) Exercise increases coronary collateral circulation in the heart.
c) Exercise prevents or delays the atheropoiesis process.
d) Exercise increases fibrinolysis.
e) Exercise causes enzyme induction, which favors cardiac aerobic metabolism as opposed to nonaerobic metabolism.

It has been observed that there are other parameters that change during a regular exercise program, such as kaolin partial thromboplastin time, which shortens, and euglobulin lysis time, which increases. If this is so, exercise could be dangerous in the untrained individual who participates on a casual or sudden basis.

Summary

Modern scientific experiments involving isotopic techniques have given validity to the study of atherosclerosis, which was originally based on scientific theory and observation. The association of cholesterol with atheropoiesis was first made in 1847 by Vogel, who found a substance in atherosclerotic lesions resembling the crystal identified by Chevreul in 1824 as cholesterol. The scientific inquiries of the next 100 years were dominated by the theory that cholesterol was responsible for atherosclerosis. This thought, crowned by the Anitschkow rabbit experiments in the early 20th century, appeared to go unchallenged. It remained for Duff to question this concept in 1935 and for others like Leary to confirm Anitschkow's theory through the use of a polarizing microscope. Further investigations unraveled the nature of the cholesterol molecule and its intermediary metabolism, which led to studies of cholesterol synthesis within the arterial wall itself. Soon it was proven that substances other than cholesterol were deposited in the arteries—substances such as phospholipids, fatty acids of various chain lengths, triglycerides, and lipoproteins.

Our investigators and many others began to search for clues that could establish an association or causal relationship between cholesterol and atheropoiesis, other than its level in the serum. Soon it was recognized that there were sex differences, hormonal differences, and species differences in the development of atheropoiesis. Thus, it was discovered that even lower levels of serum cholesterol found in control subjects in the United States were associated with heart disease in such countries as India, Pakistan, Yugoslavia, and Israel. In these countries, coronary heart disease existed in individuals with serum cholesterol levels of between 160-230 mg per cent. The demonstration by Gofman, and later Fredrickson, of the various types of lipoproteins associated with coronary heart disease suggested a lipid-carbohydrate imbalance. Thus, a shift to the study of etiologic areas other than cholesterol was realized. Our own demonstration that the histogram of the cholesterol distribution of our control and coronary subjects overlapped considerably rather than being discontinuous suggested that other etiologic agents were at work.

Considerable emphasis was placed on the clotting factor in atherosclerosis by Duguid, who extended Rokitansky's theory. It appeared that several processes were working simultaneously, that is, lipid deposition and local synthesis, fibrous deposition coupled with endothelialization, degeneration and calcification, and finally, thrombus formation.

In both 1949 and 1971, the cholesterol values obtained for the coronary and control groups revealed a significant difference ($p<.001$). The matched control group was also significantly different from the coronary group in 1949 (241 mg per cent and 286 mg per cent, respectively). The delta values in Table 6.2 reveal no statistically significant changes in the cholesterol levels in these two groups over the past 25 years, although the controls who developed C.H.D. did reveal a greater increase than the other groups.

The follow-up studies summarized in Table 6.1 revealed several important findings: (a) Serum cholesterol is of great value in predicting survival following an acute coronary episode. Those coronaries who subsequently died had a mean cholesterol value of 295 mg per cent as opposed to 248 mg per cent for the surviving coronaries. (b) Serum cholesterol was of limited value in predicting acute coronary heart episodes in the control group in this study.

There was an interesting finding regarding physique, coronary heart disease, and serum cholesterol. The levels of serum cholesterol were higher in the mesomorphs within the coronary heart disease group than in the endomorphs and ectomorphs. In comparison, the ectomorphs within the coronary group showed the lowest level of serum cholesterol of the three groups. Thus, it became evident that a similar genetic linkage might be operating to produce the coronary heart syndrome.

The Gofman finding in 1950 that lipoproteins were involved in coronary heart disease, coupled with the finding that the risk factors were controlled genetically, provided an excellent framework for the study of lipoprotein patterns and coronary heart disease. Our findings are consonant with those of other investigators who found a distribution of lipoproteins between types II and IV in heart disease patients rather than favoring type II. The importance of the lipoproteins has not been appreciated to date. They serve as an integral part of a dynamic process involving the fats and carbohydrates (via the phospholipids) in addition to being an intermediary with the proteins themselves. Study of the lipoprotein base has permitted a better understanding of clotting mechanisms, the role of phospholipids, and finally, methods of lowering serum cholesterol and triglycerides.

While measurement of phospholipids in 1949 revealed no significant differences between the control and coronary groups, the follow-up examination showed a significantly higher mean phospholipid level in the 49 deceased C.H.D. patients than in the surviving coronary group. Biserial correlations demonstrated that the level of phospholipids rose as the cholesterol level rose within the control group, but a lag existed within the coronary group. This lag could explain a change favoring procoagulation in the coronary group.

Much progress has been made in the undoing of the natural process of atheropoiesis, which has reached epidemic proportions since 1950. The fact that risk factors other than cholesterol have been implicated is not only noteworthy, but it represents the successful jump over a great hurdle in reversing and/or removing the entire process.

References

1 C. E. Bills, "Physiology of the Sterols, Including Vitamin D," *Physiol. Rev.* 15: 1-97, 1935.

2 D. Chevreul, "Note sur la Presence de la Cholesterine dans la Bile de l'Homme," *J. de Physiologie Exper.* 4: 257-260, 1824.

3 P. S. Denis, *Recherches Experimentales sur le Sang Humain, Considere à l'État Sain* (Commercy: C. F. Denis, 1830), pp. 1-358.

4 J. Vogel, *The Pathological Anatomy of the Human Body,* 1st ed. (Philadelphia: Lea and Blanchard, 1847), p. 531, 534.

5 A. Windaus, "Ueber den Gehalt Normaler und Atheromatöser Aorten an Cholesterin und Cholesterinestern," *Ztschr. F. Physiol. Chem.* 67: 174-176, 1910.

6 R. Schoenheimer, "Zur Chemie der Gesünden und der Atheroloklotischen Aorta," *Ztschr. F. Physiol. Chem.* 177: 143-157, 1928; R. Schoenheimer and W. M. Sperry, "A Micromethod for the Determination of Free and Combined Cholesterol," *J. Biol. Chem.* 106: 745-760, 1934.

7 N. Anitschkow and S. Chalatow, "Über Experimentelle Cholesterinsteatose und Ihre Bedeutung für die Enstehung Einiger Pathologischer Prozesse," *Centralbl. F. Allg. Path. U. Path. Anat.* 24: 1-9, 1913.

8 E. P. Boas, A. D. Parets, and D. Adlersberg, "Hereditary Disturbance of Cholesterol Metabolism: Factor on the Genesis of Atherosclerosis," *Am. Heart J.* 35(4): 611-622, 1948.

9 W. R. Bloor, "The Blood Lipids in Nephritis," *J. Biol. Chem.* 31: 575-583, 1917.

10 A. A. Epstein and H. Lande, "Studies on Blood Lipoids I. The Relation of Cholesterol and Protein Deficiency to Basal Metabolism," *Arch. Int. Med.* 30: 563-577, 1922.

11 S. J. Thannhauser, *Lipidoses: Disease of the Cellular Lipid Metabolism,* 1st ed. (New York: Oxford University Press, 1940), p. 41.

12 I. M. Rabinowitch, "Arteriosclerosis in Diabetes: Relationship Between Plasma Cholesterol and Arteriosclerosis; Effects of High-Carbohydrate-Low-Calorie Diet," *Ann. Int. Med.* 8:1436-1474, 1935; E. P. Joslin, W. R. Bloor, and H. Gary, "The Blood Lipids in Diabetes," *JAMA* 69: 375-378, 1917.

13 G. L. Duff, "Experimental Cholesterol Arteriosclerosis and Its Relationship to Human Arteriosclerosis," *Arch. Path.* 20: 81-123, 259-304, 1935.

14 T. Leary, "Crystalline Ester Cholesterol and Atherosclerosis," *Arch. Path.* 47: 1-28, 1949.

15 F. Reinitzer, "Beitrage zur Kenntnis des Cholesterins," *Monatschefte F. Chemie* 9: 421-441, 1888.

16 K. Bloch, "Biological Synthesis of Cholesterol," *Harvey Lectures* 48: 68-88, 1953.

17 R. Robinson, "Constitution of Cholesterol," *Nature* 130: 540-541, 1932.

18 K. Folkers, C. H. Shunk, B. O. Linn et al., "Discovery and Elucidation of Mevalonic Acid," in *Ciba Found, Symp., Biosyn. Terpenes Sterols,* (Boston: Little, Brown, 1959), pp. 119-131; L. D. Wright, "Biosynthesis of Isoprenoid Compounds," *Ann. Rev. Biochem.* 30: 525, 1961.

19 D. B. Zilversmit, "Metabolism of Arterial Lipids," in *Atherosclerosis: Proceedings of the Second International Symposium on Atherosclerosis* (New York: Springer-Verlag, 1970), pp. 35-41.

20 A. V. Chobanian and R. D. Lille, "Effects of Atherosclerosis on Lipid and Protein Synthesis in Human Aorta," in *Atherosclerosis: Proceedings of the Second International Symposium on Atherosclerosis* (New York: Springer-Verlag, 1970), pp. 282-285.

21 E. B. Smith, "The Influence of Age and Atherosclerosis on the Chemistry of Aortic Intima. 1. The Lipids," *J. Atheroscler. Res.* 5: 241-248, 1965.

22 W. A. Thomas, R. A. Florentin, S. C. Nam et al., "Plasma Lipids and Experimental Atherosclerosis," in *Atherosclerosis: Proceedings of the Second International Symposium on Atherosclerosis* (New York: Springer-Verlag, 1970), pp. 414-425.

23 F. B. Cookson, R. Altschul, and A. Fedoroff, "The Effect of Alfalfa Feeding on Serum Cholesterol and in Modifying or

Preventing Cholesterol Induced Atherosclerosis in Rabbits," *J. Atheroscler. Res.* 7: 69-81, 1969.
24 R. A. Florentin and S. C. Nam, "Dietary Induced Atherosclerosis in Miniature Swine. I. Gross and Light Microscopy Observations: Time Development and Morphological Characteristics of Lesions," *Exp. Molec. Path.* 8: 263-301, 1968.
25 R. M. O'Neal, W. J. F. Still, and W. S. Hartcroft, "Experimental Atherosclerosis in the Rat," *J. Path. Bact.* 82: 183-188, 1961.
26 O. W. Portman and M. Alexander, "Lipid Composition of Aortic Intima Plus Media and Other Tissue Fractions From Fetal and Adult Rhesus Monkeys," *Arch. Biochem. Biophys.* 117: 357-365, 1966.
27 W. A. Thomas, R. A. Florentin, S. C. Nam et al., "Pre-proliferative Phase of Atherosclerosis in Swine Fed Cholesterol," *Arch. Path.* 86: 621-643, 1968.
28 A. L. Lehninger, "The Metabolism of the Arterial Wall," in *The Arterial Wall,* Albert Lansing, ed. (Baltimore: The Williams and Wilkins Co., 1959), pp. 220-246.
29 C. Rokitansky, E. Swaine, C. H. Sieveking et al., *Manual of Pathological Anatomy,* vol. 4, trans. (Philadelphia: Blanchard and Lea, 1855), pp. 1-375.
30 F. B. Mallory, "The Infectious Lesions of Blood Vessels," in *The Harvey Lectures,* (Philadelphia: J. B. Lippincott Co., 1913), pp. 150-166.
31 E. Clark, I. Graef, and H. Chassis, "Thrombosis of the Aorta and Coronary Arteries With Special Reference to 'Fibrinoid' Lesions," *Arch. Path.* 22: 183-212, 1936.
32 J. B. Duguid and W. B. Robertson, "Mechanical Factors in Atherosclerosis," *Lancet* 1: 1205-1209, 1957.
33 S. Glagov, "Hemodynamic Factors in Localization of Atherosclerosis," *Acta. Cardiol. (Brux) Suppl.* 11: 311-337, 1965.
34 Bloor, "The Blood Lipids," pp. 575-583; W. R. Bloor and A. Knudson, "The Separate Determination of Cholesterol and Cholesterol Esters in Small Amounts of Blood," *J. Biol. Chem.* 27: 107-112, 1965.
35 C. H. Fiske and Y. Subbarow, "Colorimetric Determination of Phosphorus," *J. Biol. Chem.* 66: 375-400, 1925.
36 L, I. Abell, B. B. Levy, B. B. Brodie et al., "Simplified Method for Estimation of Total Cholesterol in Serum and Demonstration of Its Specificity," *J. Biol. Chem.* 195: 357-366, 1952.
37 Fiske and Subbarow, "Colorimetric Determination," pp. 375-400.
38 E. Van Handel and D. B. Zilversmit, "Micromethod for the Direct Determination of Serum Triglycerides," *J. Lab. Clin. Med.* 50: 152-157, 1957.
39 C. W. Frank, E. Weinblatt, and S. Shapiro, "Prognostic Implications of Serum Cholesterol in Coronary Heart Disease," in *Atherosclerosis: Proceedings of the Second International Symposium on Atherosclerosis* (New York: Springer-Verlag, 1970), pp. 390-395.
40 The Coronary Drug Project Research Group, "Clofibrate and Niacin in Coronary Heart Disease," *JAMA* 231(4): 360-381, 1975.
41 M. F. Oliver et al., "Ischaemic Heart Disease: A Secondary Prevention Trial Using Clofibrate," *Brit. Med. J.* 4: 775-784, 1971.
42 H. A. Dewar et al., "Trial of Clofibrate in the Treatment of Ischaemic Heart Disease," *Brit. Med. J.* 4: 767-775, 1971.
43 S. C. Srivastava, M. J. Smith, and H. A. Dewar, "The Effect of Atromid on Fibrinolytic Activity of Patients With Ischaemic Heart Disease and Hypercholesterolaemia," *J. Ather. Res.* 3: 640-647, 1963.
44 J. B. Gilbert and J. F. Mustard, "Some Effects of Atromid on Platelet Economy and Blood Coagulation in Man," *J. Ather. Res.* 3: 623-632, 1963.
45 M. M. Gertler, S. M. Garn, and E. F. Bland, "Age, Serum Cholesterol and Coronary Artery Disease," *Circulation* II (4): 517-522, 1950.
46 E. F. Gildea, E. Kahn, and E. B. Man, "The Relationship Between Body Build and Serum Lipids and a Discussion of These Qualities as Pyknophilic and Leptophilic Factors in the Structure of the Personality," *Am. J. Psychiat.* 92: 1247-1260, 1936; I. McQuarrie, W. R. Bloor, C. Husted, and H. A. Patterson, "Lipids of Blood Plasma in Epilepsy: a Statistical Study of Single Determinations in 100 Epileptic and 32 'Normal' Subjects," *J. Clin. Invest.* 12: 247-254, 1933; A. L. Mjassnikow, "Beitrage zur Konstitutionsforschung: Blutcholesteringehalt und Konstitution." *Ztschr. F. Klin. Med.* 105: 228-244, 1927.
47 W. H. Sheldon, S. S. Stevens, and W. B. Tucker, *The Varieties of Human Physique,* 1st ed. (New York: Harper & Bros., 1940), pp. 31-44.
48 O. F. DeLalla and J. W. Gofman, "Ultracentrifugal Analysis of Serum Lipoproteins," in *Methods of Biochemical Analysis,* D. Block, ed. (New York: New York Interscience Publishers, Inc., 1954), pp. 459-478; J. W. Gofman et al., "The Role of Lipids and Lipoproteins in Atherosclerosis," *Science* 111.2877: 166-171, 1950.
49 R. S. Lees, "Immunoassay of Plasma

Low-Density Lipoproteins," *Science* 169: 493-495, 1970.
50 R. I. Levy and D. S. Fredrickson, "Diagnosis and Management of Hyperlipoproteinemia," *Am. J. Cardiol.* 22(4): 576-583, 1968.
51 M. M. Gertler, H. E. Leetma, E. Saluste et al., "Ischemic Heart Disease: Insulin, Carbohydrate, and Lipid Interrelationships," *Circulation* 46: 103-111, 1972; M. M. Gertler, J. L. Rosenberger, H. E. Leetma, "Identification of Individuals With Covert Ischemic Thrombotic Cerebrovascular Disease: A Discriminant Function Analysis," *Stroke* 3: 764-771, 1972.
52 A. F. Salel, E. A. Amsterdam, D. T. Mason, and R. F. Zelis, "The Importance of Type IV Hyperlipoproteinemia as a Major Predisposing Metabolic Factor in Coronary Artery Disease," *Circulation* 44 (Suppl. II): 11-47, 1971.
53 E. P. Kennedy and S. B. Weiss, "Cytidine Diphosphate Choline: A New Intermediate in Lecithin Biosynthesis," *J. Am. Chem. Soc.* 77: 250-251, 1955; E. P. Kennedy and S. B. Weiss, "Functions of Cytidine Coenzymes in the Biosynthesis of Phospholipids," *J. Biol. Chem.* 222: 193-214, 1956.
54 L. Wooldridge, "Zur Gerinnung des Blutes," *Arch. F. Physiol.* Leipzig, 1883, pp. 389-393; L. C. Wooldridge, "On Intravascular Clotting," in *On the Chemistry of the Blood and Other Scientific Papers* (London: Kegan, Paul, Trench, Trubner & Co., Ltd., 1893), pp. 1-360.
55 M. J. Albrink, J. W. Meigs, and E. B. Man, "Serum Lipids, Hypertension, and Coronary Artery Disease," *Amer. J. Med.* 31: 4-23, 1961.
56 M. M. Gertler and S. M. Garn, "Lipid Interrelationship in Health and in Coronary Artery Disease," *Science* 112: 14-16, 1950.
57 E. H. Ahrens, J. Hirsch, W. Insull et al., "The Influence of Dietary Fats on Serum Lipid Levels in Man," *Lancet* 1: 943-953, 1957; A. Keys, J. T. Anderson, and F. Grande, "Serum Cholesterol Response to Changes in Diet," *Metabolism* 14: 747-758, 1965.
58 S. A. Hashim, A. Artega, and T. B. Van Itallie, "Effect of Saturated Medium-Chain Triglycerides on Serum Lipids in Man," *Lancet* 1: 1105-1109, 1960.
59 D. M. Hegsted, R. B. McGrandy, M. L. Myers, and F. J. Stare, "Quantitative Effects of Dietary Fat on Serum Cholesterol in Man," *Amer. J. Clin. Nutr.* 17: 281-295, 1965.
60 American Heart Association Monograph 18, National Diet-Heart Study Research Group, "The National Diet-Heart Study Final Report," *Circulation* 37 (Suppl. 1): 1-419, 1958; H. B. Brown, M. E. Farrand, and I. H. Page, "Design of Practical Fat-Controlled Diets, Foods, Fat Composition, and Serum Cholesterol Content," *JAMA* 196: 205-213, 1966; J. T. Anderson, F. Grande, and A. Keys, "Hydrogenated Fats in the Diet and Lipids in the Serum of Man," *J. Nutr.* 75: 388-394, 1961.
61 G. C. Chiu, "Mode of Action of Cholesterol Lowering Agents," *Arch. Int. Med.* 108: 717-732, 1961.
62 W. H. Jolins and T. R. Bates, "Quantification of the Binding Tendencies of Cholestyramine I: Effect of Structures and Added Electrolytes on the Binding of Unconjugated Bile Salt Anions," *J. Pharm. Sci.* 58(2): 179-183, 1969.
63 T. M. Parkinson, K. Gunderson, and N. A. Nelson, "Effects of Colestipol (N-26, 597), a New Bile Acid Sequestrant on Serum Lipids in Experimental Animals and Man," *Circulation* 40 (Suppl. 3): 19, 1969; G. Bazzano, M. Gray, G. Sansone-Bazzano, "Treatment of Digitalis Intoxication With a New Steroid-Binding Resin," *Clin. Res.* 18: 592, 1970.
64 D. Steinberg, "Drugs Inhibiting Cholesterol Biosynthesis, With Special Reference to Clofibrate," in *Atherosclerosis: Proceedings of the Second International Symposium on Atherosclerosis* (New York: Springer-Verlag, 1970) pp. 500-508.
65 R. Altschul, A. Hoffer, and J. D. Stephan, "Influence of Nicotinic Acid on Serum Cholesterol in Man," *Arch. Biochem.* 54: 558-559, 1955; D. Kritchevsky, M. W. Whitehouse, and E. Staple, "Oxidation of Cholesterol-26-C^{14} by Rat Liver Mitochondria: Effect of Nicotinic Acid," *J. Lipid Res.* 1: 154-158, 1960; P. Bladon, "Chemistry," in *Cholesterol, Chemistry, Biochemistry, and Pathology,* R. P. Cook, ed. (New York: Academic Press, Inc., 1958), pp. 15-115.
66 P. O. O'Reilly, "Some Clinical Aspects of Nicotinic Acid Therapy in Hypercholesterolemia," *Canad. Med. Ass. J.* 78: 402-405, 1958; O. Kraupp, E. Schnits, and H. Stromann, "Untersuchungen über den Mechanismus der Hypocholesterinamiscken Wirkung der Nicotinsaure," *Z. Ges. Exp. Med.* 129: 601-614, 1958.
67 R. Altschul and A. Hoffer, "Effect of Nicotinic Acid Upon Serum Cholesterol and Upon Basal Metabolic Rate of Young Normal Adults," *Arch. Biochem.* 73: 420-424, 1958; C. H. Duncan and M. M. Best, "Lack of Nicotinic Acid Effect on Cholesterol Metabolism of the Rat," *J. Lipid Res.* 1: 159-163, 1960.
68 O. N. Miller, J. G. Hamilton, and G. A. Goldsmith, "Investigation of the Mechanism of

Action of Nicotinic Acid on Serum Lipid Levels in Man," *Amer. J. Clin. Nutr.* 8: 480-490, 1960.
69 J. M. Merril and J. Lemley Stone, "Effect of Nicotinic Acid on Serum and Tissue Cholesterol in Rabbits," *Circulation Research* 5: 617-619, 1957.
70 O. N. Miller and J. G. Hamilton, "Nicotinic Acid and Derivatives," in *Lipid Pharmacology,* R. Paoletti, ed. (New York: Academic Press, Inc., 1964), pp. 275-298; T. A. Miettinen, "Fecal Steroid Excretion, Liver Lipids, and Conversion of Acetate and Mevalonate to Serum Cholesterol During Starvation and Nicotinic Acid Treatment," *Scand. J. Clin. Lab. Invest.* 21 (Suppl. 101): 20, 1968; W. L. Holmes, "Drugs Affecting Lipid Synthesis," in *Lipid Pharmacology,* R. Paoletti, ed. (New York: Academic Press, Inc., 1964) pp. 132-184.
71 R. L. Mason, H. M. Hunt, and L. M. Hurxthal, "Blood Cholesterol Values in Hyperthyroidism and Hypothyroidism–Their Significance," *New Eng. J. Med.* 203: 1273-1278, 1930; J. P. Peters and E. B. Man, "The Interrelations of Serum Lipids in Patients With Thyroid Disease," *J. Clin. Invest.* 22: 715-719, 1943; F. F. Foldes and A. J. Murphy, "Distribution of Cholesterol, Cholesterol Esters, and Lipid Phosphorus in Blood in Thyroid Disease," *Proc. Soc. Exp. Biol. Med.* 62: 218-223, 1946.
72 D. T. Forman, J. E. Garvin, J. E. Forestner, C. B. Taylor, "Increased Excretion of Fecal Bile Acids by an Oral Hydrophilic Colloid," *Proc. Soc. Exp. Biol. Med.* 127: 1060-1063, 1968.
73 T. M. Parkinson, "Hypolipidemic Effects of Orally Administered Dextran and Cellulose Anion Exchangers in Cockerels and Dogs," *J. Lipid Res.* 8: 24-29, 1967.
74 T. A. Miettinen, "Drugs Affecting Bile Acid and Cholesterol Excretion," in *Atherosclerosis: Proceedings of the Second International Symposium on Atherosclerosis* (New York: Springer-Verlag, 1970) pp. 508-515.
75 M. A. Eastwood and R. H. Girdwood, "Lignin, Bile-Salt Sequestrating Agent," *Lancet* II: 1170-1172, 1968.
76 P. Samuel and A. Steiner, "Effect of Neomycin on Serum Cholesterol Level in Man," *Proc. Soc. Exp. Biol. Med.* 100: 192-195, 1959; P. Samuel, C. H. Holtzman, and J. Goldstein, "Long-Term Reduction of Serum Cholesterol Levels of Patients With Atherosclerosis by Small Doses of Neomycin," *Circulation* 35: 938-945, 1967.
77 J. F. Van den Bosch and P. J. Claes, "Correlation Between the Bile-Salt Precipitating Capacity of Derivatives of Basic Antibodies and Their Cholesterol Lowering Effect in Vivo," *Progr. Biochem. Pharmacol.* 2: 97-113, 1967.
78 R. B. Moore, I. D. Frantz Jr., R. L. Varco, and H. Buchwald, "Cholesterol Dynamics After Partial Ileal Bypass," in *Atherosclerosis: Proceedings of the Second International Symposium on Atherosclerosis* (New York: Springer-Verlag, 1970) pp. 295-300.
79 S. D. Kobernick, G. Niwayama, and A. C. Zuchlewski, "The Effect of Physical Activity on Cholesterol Atherosclerosis in Rabbits," *Proc. Soc. Exp. Biol. Med.* 96: 623, 1957.

VII Biochemical Findings: The Role of Serum Uric Acid

Historical Background

The first documented description of gout is usually ascribed to Sydenham in 1686.[1] Scheele in 1776 discovered uric acid to be a constituent of a urinary stone.[2] Wollaston in 1797,[3] and Pearson in 1798,[4] found uric acid in the tophi of patients with gout. Probably the first investigator to suggest a causal relationship between gout and increased uric acid in the blood was Garrod in 1848.[5] Since Garrod's observations, a voluminous amount of literature has accumulated confirming[6] and modifying his viewpoint.[7]

The majority of gout cases are found in men in their fifth, sixth, and seventh decades of life.[8] The factors of large frame and age distribution, along with familial tendency, are common to both coronary heart disease and the gouty diathesis.[9] A causal relationship between the gouty diathesis and arteriosclerosis has been a clinical concept since the early part of this century, with such observers as Roberts noting palpitations and angina pectoris in patients with gout. Roberts also noted a proclivity towards the formation of thrombi in the veins of the lower limbs of gouty patients.[10] These astute observations were confirmed by Huchard who said, "*Gout* is to the arteries what rheumatism is to the *heart,* and this is why the presence of arterial degeneration appears to a greater degree in certain families of hereditary gout."[11]

It was this clinical suggestion—that there is an association between gout and C.H.D.—that led to this study of uric acid in the serum of coronary patients.

Biosynthesis of uric acid

Uric acid is the principal excretory product of purine catabolism, in which the purine ring is left intact. There are four purine bases from which uric acid is derived: adenine, guanine, hypoxanthine, and xanthine.[12] Guanine is deaminated by guanase to yield xanthine, which in turn is oxidized in the liver and small intestine mucosa to yield uric acid. The conversion of adenine to uric acid in man virtually does not occur. The complicated synthesis of uric acid from the purine base hypoxanthine is given below:

Carbon 2,8—derived from formate
Carbon 4,5—derived from carboxyl and methylene group of glycine
Nitrogen 7—derived from glycine
Nitrogen 1—derived from aspartic acid
Nitrogen 3,9—derived from the amide nitrogen of glutamine

The entire sequence of uric acid production is based on the reaction of L-glutamine and 5-phosphoribosyl-1-pyrophosphate, which unite under the influence of glutamine hypoxanthine $+ O_2 + H_2O_2 \rightarrow$ xanthine $+ H_2O_2$

xanthine $+ O_2 + H_2O_2 \rightarrow$ uric acid $+ H_2O_2$

phosphoribosyl pyrophosphate-amido-transferase to form 5-phosphoribosyl-1-amine. The substrates for this synthesis are natural components of the metabolic pool.[13]

The rates of uric acid turnover and production have been the subject of numerous studies with respect to gout.[14] The turnover rate is calculated by observing the amount of uric acid replaced daily in the miscible pool by newly synthesized uric acid. This is made possible by the intravenous injection of isotopic uric acid, which mixes with the subject's uric acid. The amount generally replaced on a daily basis is 41-85 per cent. The miscible pool of uric acid is obtained by calculating the amount of total uric acid in the body diluted by the labeled uric acid.[15] Various values have been obtained for normal individuals ranging from 866 mg per cent to 1,587 mg per cent (average 1,116), whereas in gouty patients the values found have been 2,000 to 31,000 mg per cent. Unfortunately, no such data are available for patients with coronary heart disease.

Heredity and hyperuricemia

What causes hyperuricemic disease? The answer is an enzyme deficiency which would account for the rise in the serum abnormalities associated with the disease.

Much progress has been made in the biochemistry relating to transferable (hereditary) deficiencies that produce hyperuricemia. There are several enzyme deficiencies now recognized in gout, such as glucose-6-phosphate deficiency, glutathione reductase deficiency, and hypoxanthine-guanine phosphoribosyl transferase deficiency (as seen in the Lesch-Nyhan syndrome).[16]

The question of the genetic pattern of hyperuricemia appears divided into two schools of thought: an autosomal dominant gene theory and a polygenic trait theory. The dominant gene theory tends to predominate in studies that are isolated in terms of several generations of particular families and/or race.[17] The polygenic trait theory is a more probable explanation of hereditary pattern in heterogeneous populations, as in siblings of gouty patients.[18] Enzyme deficiencies as in the Lesch-Nyhan syndrome are explained as X-linked conditions.[19] The evidence assembled in this study does not warrant a statement in favor of any one theory of genetic transference of hyperuricemia.

In an interesting study of the Maori living on different islands around New Zealand, a high degree of hyperuricemia as well as diabetic abnormalities was noted. But the highest percentage was found in the Maori who actually lived in New Zealand.[20] Although genetic factors contributed to the high incidence of these diseases, the study also stressed that the high calorie and fat diets and the alcohol that New Zealand's Maori were exposed to may have brought out the predisposition and been responsible for the highest observed rates of all the Maori studied. Thus, both genetic and environmental factors are implicated in gout and diabetes mellitus.

Uric Acid and Associated Diseases

The term gout was probably derived from the French word "gout," meaning taste or flavor. Historically, the gouty patient has been portrayed as a fat, lethargic male who is generally a gourmand. The high degree of correlation we found between serum uric acid and endomorphy (see Table 7.1) confirms this impression. Other investigators have reported similar findings.[21]

It is only natural to extend the correlation between uric acid and obesity to uric acid and diabetes, since obesity and diabetes are often associated. Robert Whytt, in 1768, was the first to suggest an association between diabetes mellitus and gouty arthritis.[22] A review of the literature indicates that at least 20 per cent of gouty patients have chemical diabetes, with some reports as high as 50 per cent.[23] On the other hand, Beckett found only eight cases of gout in 1,000 diabetics,[24] and Whitehouse reported it in 1.6 per cent of the diabetics he studied.[25] These findings confirm the observations of Bartels and Ishmael, who noted that the clinical manifestation of gout precedes diabetes.[26] Such findings are not unusual in light of the observation that diabetes has an ameliorating effect on gout due to the increased excretion of uric acid that accompanies diabetes.[27]

While a relationship between uric acid and diabetes has not been established, it has been theorized that a deviation in the synthesis or degradation of uric acid may lead to the production of alloxan, a substance that has been shown to produce diabetes through the destruction of pancreatic beta cells. Since uric acid and alloxan are so similar, all that would be required is the elimination of one urea molecule. Another theory takes into account the fact that uric acid is a potent inhibitor of monoamine oxidase.[28] This information, coupled with Cegrell's observation that the inhibition of monoamine oxidase may affect the biogenic amine levels in the pancreatic beta cell,[29] could mean that high levels of uric acid also produce a nonactive insulin (proinsulin) or a reduced amount of insulin secondary to fatigue of the beta cells.

The role of uric acid in coronary heart disease may also be related to the high incidence of diabetes mellitus found among heart disease patients.[30] Varying amounts of the intermediates of purine synthesis, among other factors, may be accumulating in C.H.D. patients, which could either diminish or increase the activity of cyclic adenosine monophosphate (CAMP) available for insulin regulatory purposes. It is probable, however, that the relationship between uric acid and diabetes mellitus is related to other variables, particularly obesity, since the concomitance of obesity in gouty and diabetic patients is very high.[31]

Reports in the literature indicate that as many as 85 per cent of patients with gout

Table 7.1 Coefficients of correlation between serum uric acid and Sheldonian classifications in the coronary and control groups

Classification	Coronary group	Control group
Endomorphy	0.29 ± .10*	0.38 ± .08*
Mesomorphy	−0.05 ± .10	0.23 ± .08*
Ectomorphy	−0.13 ± .10	−0.29 ± .08

*Significant correlation

have hypertriglyceridemia,[32] and that as many as 82 per cent of patients with hypertriglyceridemia have coexistent hyperuricemia.[33] These same findings were made in our laboratory. After feeding a uricase inhibitor (oxonic acid) to rabbits, there was a rise in serum uric acid that was paralleled by a rise in triglycerides. When uric acid levels were permitted to return to normal, the serum triglyceride levels also returned to normal. Similar results were observed among male subjects. Lower triglyceride levels were found in men with serum uric acid levels under 6.5 mg per cent than in men with uric acid levels above 6.5 mg per cent.

The reason for this is not entirely clear. But it would be reasonable to suggest that the rise in serum uric acid levels affects insulin secretion, which in turn may produce excessive esterification of L-alpha glycerol levels with free fatty acids, thus producing an increase in triglyceride levels.[34] This is supported by other investigators' observations that type IV lipoproteinemia, which is seen in diabetes mellitus as well as C.H.D. and ITCVD (ischemic thrombotic cerebrovascular disease), is comprised of hypertriglyceridemia, normal or moderately elevated cholesterol, and hyperuricemia.[35]

There are multiple causes for hyperuricemia. Among them are: (a) diet, when there is heavy ingestion of uric acid precursors;[36] (b) increased synthesis, such as in gout; (c) decreased excretion due to renal failure;[37] or (d) a combination of these factors. Other causes of hyperuricemia are (a) increased cellular breakdown, from lymphoproliferative diseases such as leukemia, or secondary to chemotherapy from cytotoxic drugs,[38] and (b) diuretics such as chlorothiazides.[39] Patients given chlorothiazide therapy exhibit not only an increase in uric acid level but also an increase in abnormal glucose tolerance response. When the chlorothiazide therapy is discontinued, the uric acid levels tend to drop. It is noteworthy that glucose tolerance tests and immunoreactive insulin levels tend to normalize during the return of uric acid levels to normal. Excessive urate binding to plasma proteins has also been implicated.

Clinical Observations

A comparison of the 1949 serum uric acid values for the original coronary, matched control, and unmatched control groups is given in Figure 7.1. The average level of serum uric acid in the coronary heart disease group was significantly higher than in the matched control group. Forty-eight per cent of the coronary patients had levels of 5.0 or over, compared with 41 per cent of the matched controls. At levels of 6.0 or over the difference was much greater, or 22 per cent of the coronary group as opposed to 6 per cent of the matched controls.

Figure 7.1 Frequency distribution of uric acid in coronary heart disease group, unmatched control group, and matched control group. Note that 22 per cent of the individuals within the coronary group had serum uric acid values greater than 6.0 mg. %, while only 6 per cent of the unmatched or matched control groups had serum uric acid values greater than 6.0 mg. %.

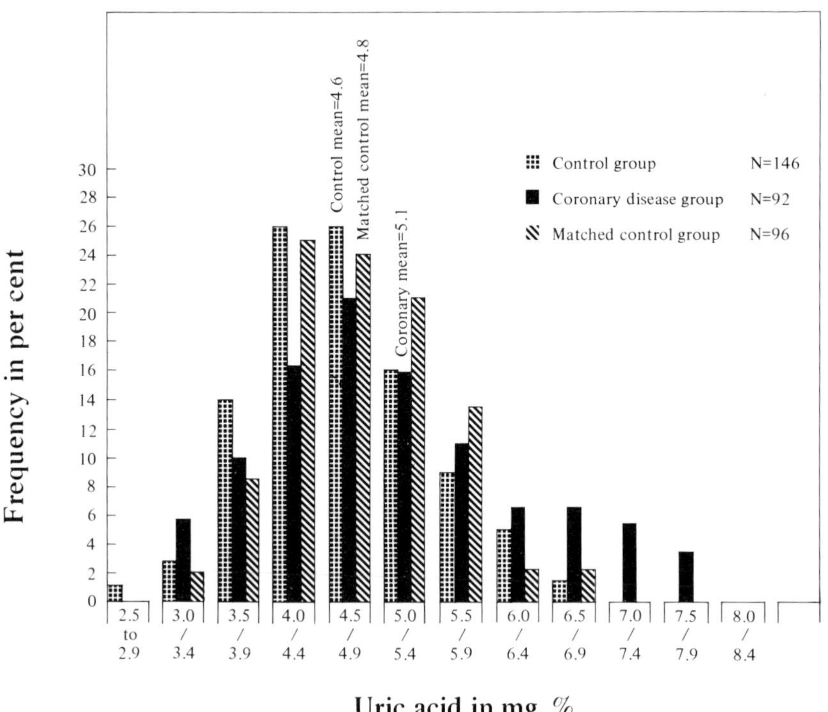

Permission to reproduce granted by Harvard University Press and M. M. Gertler, P. D. White, *Coronary Heart Disease in Young Adults* (Cambridge: Harvard University Press, 1954), p. 119. Copyright 1954 by The Commonwealth Fund.

For the 1949 determination, both the coronary and matched control groups were subdivided by age, and the average uric acid levels were compared. Differences in age did not seem to change the value, however. This contrasts with the change in serum total cholesterol, which showed a small but significant rise with age in both groups.

Uric acid in the surviving coronary group

The 1949 data concerning the relationship of serum uric acid values to subsequent survival permit some hypothesizing. The surviving coronary group had a significantly lower mean uric acid level in 1949 than did the 71 expired individuals from the original coronary group. (See Table 7.2.) This may reaffirm the contention that an increased serum uric acid level does contribute to the acceleration of existing coronary heart

Table 7.2 Comparison of 1949 uric acid values of coronary and control groups

	Number	Mean ± S.D.	t	p<
Coronary group	93	5.03 ± 1.15	2.80	.01
Control group	146	4.67 ± 0.83		
Surviving coronary group	21	4.57 ± 1.02	−2.15	.05
Expired coronary group	71	5.18 ± 1.17		

Table 7.3 Correlations with serum uric acid in coronary and control groups (1949)

Variable	Coronary group (92)	Control group (140)
Height	.10 ± .10	−.07 ± .08
Weight	.30 ± .08*	.23 ± .10*
Ponderal index	−.37 ± .07*	−.22 ± .10*

*Significant correlation

disease. The lower uric acid values of the surviving coronary group may be one of the factors that promoted longer survival after the onset of the disease.

Uric acid and morphological characteristics

Since it had been shown that the highest levels of serum total cholesterol occur in the mesomorphs[40] who experience coronary heart disease, we decided to study the relationship between serum uric acid and morphological characteristics in both the matched control and coronary groups. Consequently, coefficients of correlation were determined between serum uric acid and height, weight, and ponderal index.

Certain information may be gathered from the coefficients of correlation seen in Table 7.3: (a) There was an insignificant correlation between uric acid and height in the coronary and matched control groups. (b) There was a significant correlation between uric acid and weight for both groups. (c) There were significant correlations between ponderal index and uric acid in both groups.

Thus, linear measurement, per se, is unrelated to serum uric acid. But as actual weight and relative body mass of an individual increase, as reflected in the ponderal index, the serum uric acid has a tendency to rise. Such rough estimates of physique suggest that dominant ectomorphs would have lower levels of uric acid in the serum, while dominant mesomorphs and endomorphs would have higher levels of uric acid. To evaluate these suggestions more critically, correlations were made between the Sheldonian classifications and serum uric acid. These correlations, it was thought, would be more meaningful than the correlations of uric acid to height, weight, and ponderal index, because body mass could be defined more accurately (see Table 7.1).

The results revealed a significant correlation between endomorphy and uric acid in the coronary group, while those coronary group members classified as ectomorphs showed no significant correlation. The distributions shown in Table 7.4 support this observation. The levels of serum uric acid decrease from a high level in the endomorphic

Table 7.4 Serum uric acid, by physiques, in coronary heart disease group of 92 males and unmatched control group of 146 males

Physique	Number	Serum uric acid (mg. %)	
		Range	Mean ± S.E.
Endomorphs			
Coronary	23	3.6-7.6	5.61 ± .23
Control	51	3.1-6.9	4.87 ± .12
Difference			*
Mesomorphs			
Coronary	41	3.2-7.7	4.98 ± .18
Control	34	3.6-5.4	4.59 ± .09
Difference			ns
Ectomorphs			
Coronary	9	3.9-6.1	4.80 ± .23
Control	34	2.9-5.8	4.34 ± .12
Difference			ns
Mid-range			
Coronary	19	3.2-7.8	5.01 ± .27
Control	27	3.8-6.2	4.65 ± .12
Difference			ns

*Highly significant

subjects to a low level in the ectomorphic subjects. The difference is significant in both the C.H.D. and control groups. This confirms, in general, the negative correlation between serum uric acid and ponderal index. It also adds support to the relationship between hyperuricemia, endomorphy, and coronary heart disease.

Correlations between uric acid and other risk factors

The coefficients of correlation between serum uric acid, cholesterol, and phospholipids were determined from the 1949 data as well as the 1971 follow-up, with the addition of triglycerides. The following information may be gathered from the results of the 1949 data: (a) The correlation between uric acid and cholesterol was insignificant for both the coronary and control groups, and (b) there was an insignificant correlation between uric acid and phospholipids for the coronary group, while there was a significant positive correlation between serum uric acid and phospholipids in the control group. The 1971 correlations revealed the following information: (a) There was a significant correlation between serum uric acid and all three lipids, cholesterol, phospholipids, and triglycerides in the control group; (b) as in the 1949 data, the surviving coronary group showed an insignificant relationship between uric acid, cholesterol, and phospholipids; and (c) the correlation between uric acid and triglycerides in this group showed a relationship similar to the control group, although it did not reach statistical significance due to the limited sample size (see Tables 7.5 and 7.6).

Table 7.5 Coefficients of correlation in the coronary and control groups for 1949 serum uric acid values

Variable	Coronary group (66)	p<	Control group (146)	p<
Cholesterol	–0.06	ns	0.12	ns
Phospholipids	–0.04	ns	0.19	.05

Table 7.6 Coefficients of correlation in the coronary and control groups for 1971 uric acid values

Variable	Coronary group (19)	p<	Control group (112)	p<
Cholesterol	0.11	ns	0.19	.05
Phospholipids	–0.06	ns	0.26	.01
Triglycerides	0.38	.01	0.33	.001

Table 7.7 Coefficients of correlation with uric acid in healthy men and women over 65 years of age

Variable	Men (38)	Women (91)
Cholesterol	0.49 ± .08*	0.00 ± .10
Lipid phosphorus	0.52 ± .08*	–0.10 ± .10
Sf molecules	0.37 ± .10*	0.12 ± .11
Ponderal index	–0.26 ± 1.4	–0.25 ± .19*

*p<.001

The correlation data seen in these tables provide further support for the relationship between serum uric acid and serum triglycerides as observed in our studies of rabbits and man. No explanation is available for the significant correlation of phospholipids and uric acid in the control group and the lack of significance seen in the coronary group.

An interesting study concerning metabolic factors associated with C.H.D. was conducted in Busselton, Western Australia, and revealed that serum uric acid levels possessed the most discriminating power (p<.05). But this discrimination was linked through abnormalities of lipids, such as triglycerides, rather than through a direct correlation with C.H.D.[41]

Serum uric acid in older individuals

A study conducted in 1952 by this research team indicated that the average serum uric acid level in men and women over the age of 65 was within normal limits, or 4.96±.14 and 4.55±.10, respectively.[42] The correlations between serum uric acid and other variables were impressive in that the two groups differed considerably (see Table 7.7). It was shown that uric acid levels were correlated with lipids in men but not in women. In addition, the lower ponderal indices, which are a reflection of endomorphy, were significantly correlated with elevated uric acid in women and pointed to the same trend in

Table 7.8 Mean differences in uric acid in control and coronary groups between 1949 and 1971 determinations

	Number	1949 Mean ± S.D.	1971 Mean ± S.D.	Mean differences	p<
Surviving controls with C.H.D.	14	4.57 ± .94	6.06 ± 1.39	1.49 ± 1.75	.01
Surviving controls without C.H.D.	100	4.67 ± .82	5.95 ± 1.16	1.27 ± 1.15	.001
Surviving coronary group	19	4.57 ± 1.02	6.25 ± .99	1.75 ± 1.16	.001

men. Such data emphasized the importance of the association between uric acid and lipids in men and reaffirmed the relationship between endomorphy and hyperuricemia previously shown in younger individuals. Thus, there does not appear to be a uric acid-age relationship.[43] However, uric acid does appear to rise during the peak growth periods from the early teens to the early 20s and then level off through the ninth decade of life.

The mean difference for serum uric acid from 1949 to 1971 in the surviving coronary group, the surviving controls who developed C.H.D. subsequent to the original exam in 1949, and the surviving controls who did not develop C.H.D. indicates a significant increase in this variable with age. At first glance this appears to be in direct contrast to other observations that demonstrate an absence of uric acid increase after the early 20s. Yet, there are great differences between the ways these studies were conducted. The study concerned with uric acid in individuals over the age of 65 was essentially a static study in which uric acid determinations were made at one time for a single group. The determinations of uric acid for the present study group reflected a single group observed over a span of 25 years. In addition, there may be some relationship between this increase with age and the methods employed over the years to determine serum uric acid, as well as differences in diet resulting in changes in natural and physiological processes.

Table 7.8 shows the over-all elevated value of serum uric acid in the three groups. However, there is no demonstrable statistical difference between them for 1971 values, as compared to the significant difference in uric acid between the control and coronary groups in 1949.

Summary

Uric acid was studied in the coronary and control groups because of the past clinical suggestion of an association between gout and coronary heart disease. At the time of the original study, it was found that the level of serum uric acid was significantly higher in the coronary heart disease group than in the matched control group. The follow-up study revealed that the surviving members of the coronary group had a significantly lower serum uric acid level in 1949 than the deceased coronary group, thus affirming the contention that increased levels of uric acid contribute to the acceleration of existing coronary heart disease.

When body type was examined in relation to the level of uric acid, serum uric acid was found to be significantly correlated with weight and ponderal index. Correlations were made between the Sheldonian classifications and serum uric acid, revealing that endomorphs had the highest uric acid levels and ectomorphs the lowest.

The consideration of uric acid as a risk factor is supported by the significant correlations with triglycerides and diabetes mellitus. These correlations suggest that as a risk factor, uric acid operates through its effect on insulin and triglycerides and not in relationship with serum cholesterol. This was further strengthened by nonsignificant correlations between serum uric acid and phospholipids in the diseased group, whereas the correlation was significant in the control group.

References

1 T. Sydenham, *Tractatus de Podagra et Hydrope* (Geneva: S. de Tournes, 1686), pp. 1-147.

2 K. W. Scheele, "Examen Chemicum Calculi Urinarii," *Opuscala* II: 73, 1776.

3 W. H. Wollaston, "On Gouty and Urinary Concretions," *Phil. Tr. Roy. Soc.* London, 87: 386-400, 1797.

4 G. Pearson, "Experiments and Observations Tending to Show the Composition and Properties of Urinary Concretions," *Phil. Tr. Roy. Soc.* London, 88: 15-34, 1798.

5 A. B. Garrod, "Observations on Certain Pathological Conditions of the Blood and Urine in Gout, Rheumatism and Bright's Disease," *Medico-Chir. Tr.* London, 31: 83-97, 1848.

6 E. P. Jordan and D. Gaston, "The Blood Uric Acid in Disease," *J. Clin. Invest.* 11: 747-752, 1932; B. M. Jacobson, "The Uric Acid in the Serum of Gouty and Non-Gouty Individuals: Its Determination by Folin's Recent Method and Its Significance in the Diagnosis of Gout," *Ann. Int. Med.* 11: 1277-1295, 1938.

7 M. A. Schnitker and A. B. Richter, "Nephritis in Gout," *Am. J. Med. Sci.* 192: 241-252, 1936; D. Adlersberg, E. Grishman, and H. Sobotka, "Uric Acid Partition in Gout in Hepatic Disease," *Arch. Int. Med.* 60: 101-120, 1942.

8 C. Scudamore, *A Treatise on the Nature and Cure of Gout*, 4th ed. (London: Longman, Hurst, Rees, Orme, and Brown, 1823), pp. 1-711.

9 C. J. Smyth, C. W. Cotterman, and R. H. Freyberg, "The Genetics of Gout and Hyperuricemia–An Analysis of Nineteen Families," *J. Clin. Invest.* 27: 749-759, 1948; H. Huchard, *Traité Clinique des Maladies du Coeur et de l'Aorta,* 3 vols., 3rd ed. (Paris: O. Doin, 1899-1903).

10 W. Roberts, "Gout," in *A System of Medicine by Many Writers,* T. C. Allbutt and H. D. Rolleston, eds. (London: Macmillan, 1905-1911), pp. 155-195.

11 Huchard, *Traité Clinique,* vol. 1, 1899, p. 397.

12 H. R. Mahler and E. H. Cordes, *Biological Chemistry* (New York: Harper & Row, 1966), p. 718.

13 H. Wiener, "Über Synthetische Bidung der Harnsaure in Tierkorper," *Beitr. Chem. Physiol. Path.* 2: 42, 1902; F. W. Barnes and R. Schoenheimer, "On Biological Synthesis of Purines and Pyrimidines," *J. Biol. Chem.* 51: 123-139, 1943.

14 J. D. Benedict, P. H. Forsham, and D. W. Stetten Jr., "The Metabolism of Uric Acid in the Normal and Gouty Human Studies With the Aid of Isotopic Uric Acid," *J. Biol. Chem.* 181: 183-193, 1949; J. E. Seegmiller, A. I. Grayzel, L. Laster, and L. Liddle, "Uric Acid Production in Gout," *J. Clin. Invest.* 40: 1304-1314, 1961.

15 J. D. Benedict, P. H. Forsham, M. Roche, S. Soloway, and D. W. Stetten Jr., "The Effect of Salicylates and Adrenocorticotropic Hormone Upon the Miscible Pool of Uric Acid in Gout," *J. Clin. Invest.* 29: 1104-1111, 1950; Seegmiller et al., "Uric Acid Production in Gout," pp. 1304-1314.

16 J. E. Seegmiller, "Diseases of Purine and Pyrimidine Metabolism" in *Duncan's Diseases of Metabolism,* P. K. Bondy, ed. (Philadelphia: Saunders, 1969), p. 516; W. K. Long, "Glutathione Reductase in Red Blood Cells. Variant Associated With Gout," *Science* 155: 712-716, 1967; J. E. Seegmiller, R. M. Rosenbloom, and W. N. Kelly, "An Enzyme Defect Associated With a Sex-Linked Human Neurological Disorder and Excessive Purine Synthesis," *Science* 155: 1682-1684, 1967.

17 C. J. Smyth, R. M. Stecher, and W. Q. Wolfson, "Genetic and Endocrine Determinants of the Plasma Urate Level," *Science* 108: 514-515, 1948; R. M. Stecher, A. H. Hersh, and W. M. Solomon, "The Heredity of Gout and Its Relationship to Familial Hyperuricemia," *Ann. Int. Med.* 31: 595-614, 1949.

18 M. Hauge and B. Harvald, "Heredity in Gout and Hyperuricemia," *Acta Med. Scand.* 152: 257, 1955; E. M. O'Brien, T. A. Burch, and J. J. Bunim, "Genetics of Hyperuricemia in Blackfoot and Pima Indians," *Ann. Rheum. Dis.* 25: 117-123, 1966.

19 S. L. Shapiro, G. L. Sheppard Jr., F. E. Dreifuss, and D. S. Newcombe, "X-Linked Recessive Inheritance of a Syndrome of Mental Retardation With Hyperuricemia," *Proc. Soc. Exper. Biol. Med.* 122: 609-612, 1966.

20 I. A. M. Prior, B. S. Rose, H. P. B. Harvey, and S. Davidson, "Hyperuricemia, Gout and Diabetic Abnormality in Polynesian People," *Lancet* 1: 333-338, 1966.

21 R. M. Acheson and C. D. Florey, "Body Weight, ABO Blood Groups, and Altitude of Domicile as Determinants of Serum Uric Acid in Military Recruits in Four Countries," *Lancet* 2: 391-394, 1969; R. M. Acheson and W. M. O'Brien, "Dependence of Serum Uric Acid on Haemoglobin and Other Factors in the General Population," *Lancet* 2: 777-778, 1966.

22 R. Whytt, *The Works of Robert Whytt* (Edinburgh: Beckett, 1768), p. 707.

23 J. B. Herman, "Gout and Diabetes," *Metabolism* 7: 703-706, 1958; C. Bernheim, E. Martin, H. Ott, and G. Zahnd, "Goutte et Diabete," *J. Clin. Diabet. Hotel Dieu* 10: 53, 1969; W. M. Mikkelsen, "The Possible Association of Hyperuricemia and/or Gout With Diabetes Mellitus," *Arthritis Rheum.* 8: 853-864, 1965.

24 A. G. Beckett and J. G. Lewis, "Gout and Serum Uric Acid in Diabetes Mellitus," *Quart. J. Med.* 29: 443-458, 1960.

25 F. W. Whitehouse and W. J. Cleary, "Diabetes Mellitus in Patients With Gout," *JAMA* 197: 113-116, 1966.

26 E. C. Bartels, M. C. Balodimos, and L. R. Corn, "The Association of Gout and Diabetes Mellitus," *Med. Clin. N. Amer.* 44: 433-438, 1960; W. K. Ishmael, J. N. Owens, R. W. Payne, and M. D. Honick, "Diabetes Mellitus in Patients With Gouty Arthritis," *JAMA* 190: 396-398, 1964.

27 A. G. Beckett et al., "Gout and Serum Uric Acid in Diabetes Mellitus," 1960; J. Padova, A. Patchefsky, G. Onesti, G. Faludi, and G. Bendersky, "The Effect of Glucose Loads on Renal Uric Acid Excretion in Diabetic Patients," *Metabolism* 13: 507-512, 1964.

28 L. Galzigna, G. Maina, and G. Rumney, "Role of L-Ascorbic Acid in the Reversal of the Monoamine Oxidase Inhibitor by Caffeine," *J. Pharm. Pharmac.* 23: 303-305, 1971.

29 L. Cegrell, B. Falk, and B. Hellman, "Monoaminergic Mechanisms in the Endocrine Pancreas" in *The Structure and Metabolism of the Pancreatic Islets,* S. E. Brolin, B. Hellman, and H. Knutson, eds. (New York: The Macmillan Co., 1964), p. 429.

30 M. M. Gertler, H. E. Leetma, E. Saluste, J. L. Rosenberger, and R. G. Guthrie, "Ischemic Heart Disease: Insulin, Carbohydrate, and Lipid Interrelationships," *Circulation* 46: 103-111, 1972.

31 J. A. Boyle, M. McKiddie, K. D. Buchanan, M. K. Jasani et al., "Diabetes Mellitus and Gout. Blood Sugar and Plasma Insulin Responses to Oral Glucose in Normal Weight and Overweight and Gouty Patients," *Ann. Rheum. Dis.* 28: 374-379, 1969.

32 D. Berkowitz, "Gout, Hyperlipidemia, and Diabetes Mellitus Interrelationships," *JAMA* 197: 77-80, 1966; K. A. Barlow, "Hyperlipidemia in Primary Gout," *Metabolism* 17: 289-299, 1968.

33 D. Berkowitz, "Blood Lipids and Uric Acid Interrelationships," *JAMA* 190: 856-858, 1964.

34 S. B. Weiss and E. P. Kennedy, "The Enzyme Synthesis of Triglycerides," *J. Am. Chem. Soc.* 78: 3550, 1956.

35 P. H. Schreibman, D. E. Wilson, and R. A. Arky, "Familial Type IV Hyperlipoproteinemia," *New Eng. J. Med.* 281: 981-985, 1969; D. S. Fredrickson, R. I. Levy, and R. S. Lees, "Fat Transport in Lipoproteins–An Integrated Approach to Mechanisms and Disorders," *New Eng. J. Med.* 276: 34-44, 1967.

36 G. E. Plante, J. Durivage, and G. Lemieux, "Renal Excretion of Hydrogen in Primary Gout," *Metabolism* 17: 377-385, 1968.

37 A. Kasanen, V. Kallio, and T. Markanen, "On Serum Uric Acid and Endogenic Uric Acid Clearance in Renal Failure," *Acta Med. Scand.* 160: 503-507, 1958.

38 A. Rastagar and S. D. Thier, "The Physiologic Approach to Hyperuricemia," *New Eng. J. Med.* 286: 470-476, 1972.

39 L. A. Healy and A. P. Hall, "The Epidemiology of Hyperuricemia," *Bull. Rheum. Dis.* 20: 600-603, 1970; R. H. Schwab, J. K. Perloff, and R. L. Porus, "Chlorothiazide-Induced Gout and Diabetes, Their Sequential Occurrence in the Same Patient," *Arch. Int. Med.* 3: 465-469, 1963.

40 M. M. Gertler, S. M. Garn, and J. Lerman, "The Interrelationships of Serum Cholesterol, Cholesterol Esters and Phospholipids in Health and in Coronary Artery Disease," *Circulation* 2: 204-214, 1950.

41 T. A. Weborn, D. J. A. Jenkins, G. N. Cumpston et al., "Metabolic Factors Associated With Coronary Heart Disease in Busselton Males," in *Atherosclerosis: Proceedings of the Second International Symposium on Atherosclerosis* (New York: Springer-Verlag, 1970) pp. 369-373.

42 M. M. Gertler and B. S. Oppenheimer, "Serum Uric Acid Levels in Men and Women Past the Age of 65 Years," *J. of Geront.* 8: 465-471, 1953.

43 W. M. Mikkelsen, H. J. Dodge, and H. Valkenberg, "The Distribution of Serum Uric Acid Values in a Population Unselected as to Gout or Hyperuricemia, Tecumseh, Michigan 1959-1960," *Am. J. Med.* 39: 242-251, 1965.

VIII Diet: Cholesterol Ingestion and Atherosclerosis

The relationship between diet and atheropoiesis and, hence, coronary heart disease has been a topic of discussion and investigation for many years. Many physicians believe that diet is causally related to coronary heart disease, though there is much evidence that does not support this. Present-day evidence suggests that dietary factors can influence the rate of development of coronary heart disease. This hypothesis will be evaluated, and studies done in the course of these investigations will be cited. In addition, the theoretical concepts relating dietary fats to coagulation-dietary relationships will offer some support to the dietary influence theory and suggest some mechanistic associations between diet and coronary heart disease.

A major topic of investigation in this study was the relation of cholesterol ingestion to atherosclerosis. Claims have been made that atherosclerosis occurs less frequently in countries where cholesterol is ingested in smaller quantities than in countries where the amount of cholesterol ingested is greater.[1] Such specific questions will be discussed later in the chapter. The evidence supporting the influence of diet on atheropoiesis stems not only from clinical observations and investigations but also from large-scale national and international epidemiological and experimental studies. The over-all evidence is not entirely conclusive for any single dietary area; except perhaps where total fat and, particularly, excessive saturated fat intake is involved. But the question of diet and atherosclerogenesis is not merely one of the relationship between fats and serum cholesterol and, hence, atheropoiesis. It is, rather, an encompassing concept involving fats and carbohydrates and perhaps proteins as well. In addition to these relationships, one must consider the over-all caloric intake as well as cholesterol itself.

There are data indicating that excessive cholesterol feedings may produce atherosclerosis in dogs[2] and rabbits.[3] While some investigators have accepted such evidence as applicable to man,[4] others are reluctant to do so because (a) the amount of cholesterol employed in these experiments far exceeds the highest physiological level of ingestion by man, and (b) the lesions are distributed mainly in the distal arteries and, to a lesser degree, involve the coronary arteries. Duff has questioned whether the disease processes in man and rabbits are comparable.[5] In addition, alteration in the metabolism has to be superimposed in some animals.[6]

Through the use of deuterium-labeled and ^{14}C-labeled precursors, it has been demonstrated that cholesterol may be synthesized in pigeons, mice, and rats.[7] It has also been shown that cholesterol is synthesized from amino acids (such as leucine and alanine), acetic acid, mevalonic acid, and fatty acids (such as myristic and butyric acids).[8] In all probability, similar mechanisms of synthesis exist in man, despite the failure to demonstrate all of them as yet. In our study, analysis of the dietary records of the coronary and control groups revealed no correlation between the amount of these substances in the diet and the level of serum cholesterol.

A general relationship has been claimed to exist between atherosclerosis and nutrition on the grounds that atherosclerosis occurs more frequently in individuals who are overweight,[9] and that it declines in the population during periods of famine.[10] Whether or not there is a causal relationship between atherosclerosis and degree of nutrition cannot be determined from this evidence alone.

The relationship between weight and coronary heart disease was discussed in Chapter V, where it was shown that in the present study the coronary patients were not overweight when compared to the controls. Walker, who summarized the effects of dietary restriction on serum lipids, demonstrated that weight reduction reduces serum lipids.[11] Recent evidence also supports this viewpoint.[12]

Sources of Cholesterol in Atherosclerosis

It is well known that serum cholesterol is frequently elevated in coronary heart disease. It is also well known that atherosclerotic plaques, which are responsible for coronary heart disease, contain more cholesterol and cholesterol esters than the surrounding arterial tissue. These two factors—hypercholesterolemia and cholesterol deposition—are thought to be causally related. The reason for this belief is that when cholesterol is ingested in large quantities it produces an elevated serum cholesterol. It is believed that an elevated serum cholesterol will eventually produce atherosclerosis. Chapter VI reviewed two aspects of evidence that oppose these contentions: (a) The serum cholesterol distribution curves of both the control group and coronary heart disease group are not discontinuous and overlap to a considerable degree, and (b) the interrelations of the other lipids such as phospholipids may be as important in the deposition of cholesterol as cholesterol itself. Furthermore, no one has demonstrated beyond a reasonable doubt in human subjects that the source of the cholesterol in the atherosclerotic plaque is solely dietary. The evidence is still lacking to support the viewpoint that a major portion of plaque cholesterol is derived from exogenous cholesterol.[13] There is also evidence that does not support the theory that cholesterol is synthesized in the plaque to a degree sufficient to produce definite atherosclerotic lesions.[14] Therefore, one is forced to conclude that both endogenous and exogenous sources play a definite role in plaque development. Studies concerned with the source of lipids within the arterial wall and plaque indicate that phospholipids are derived primarily from local synthesis in the foam cells.[15] In the experimental animal, cholesterol infiltrates into the wall in virtually direct proportion to the level of serum cholesterol.[16] It is doubtful whether similar observations can be made when dealing with physiologic levels of cholesterol rather than unusual pathologic challenges. Thus, conclusions concerning arterial lipid accumulation, biosynthesis, and influx in man cannot be ventured until further data become available. It is interesting that at any lipid level, the level of the mean blood pressure has been shown to influence the amount of cholesterol deposited in the arterial wall.[17] Thus, the field of inquiry broadens and is not limited to diet alone.

Relation of ingested cholesterol to serum cholesterol

Because of claims that increased ingestion of cholesterol produces an elevated level of serum cholesterol, it was decided at the time of the original study to (a) determine the average amount of cholesterol ingested per week for both the coronary heart disease group prior to infarction and the control group, and (b) correlate the amount of cholesterol ingested with the level of cholesterol in the serum for these two groups.

The control group, on the average, ingested significantly more cholesterol than the coronary heart disease group (18 per cent more), but had significantly less cholesterol in the serum than the coronary group (224.2 mg per cent versus 286.5 mg per cent). It is clear that in the coronary group, in spite of the lower average ingestion of cholesterol, both the individuals who ingested either large quantities or small quantities still had an average serum total cholesterol significantly higher than that of the control group.

It was apparent that a factor or factors in addition to ingested cholesterol were important. This conclusion gained further support from the insignificant coefficients of correlation between the amount of ingested cholesterol and the level of serum cholesterol for both groups: +.05 for the unmatched control group, -.09 for the coronary heart disease group. Thus, there was practically no correlation between the amount of cholesterol in the serum and exogenous cholesterol. The evidence in 1949 pointed to endogenous sources of cholesterol as an additional source and, hence, as an important contributor to coronary heart disease. This theory has received support in recent publications; studies by Kang-Jey Ho and co-workers indicate that cholesterol synthesized in the liver, skin, and small intestine finds its way into the metabolic pool, including the blood plasma.[18] This was described in an elegant study by Goodman.[19] It is interesting to note that starvation will not affect synthesis in the extrahepatic areas. Since the liver is the major source of endogenous cholesterol, it may be concluded that dietary cholesterol could indirectly affect the over-all content of the cholesterol pool. However, the facts in human studies do not fit the conclusions from animal experiments, but rather suggest that although the cholesterol pool can be decreased by exogenous sources, the level of serum cholesterol is not correlated with the cholesterol pool.

Relation of serum cholesterol to atherosclerosis

Moreton brought out an interesting theory, supported by experimental evidence, on the etiology of atherosclerosis. He demonstrated that fat particles (chylomicrons) appearing in normal plasma during alimentary hyperlipemia are of colloidal size and, upon ultracentrifugation, are shown to consist mainly of neutral fats and lipid phosphorus in addition to minute quantities of cholesterol and other substances.[20] The micelles were later categorized by Gofman et al. as Sf 20-400 molecules.[21] Moreton suggested that the cause of atherosclerosis in humans is the accumulation of showers of chylomicrons in the arteries over a long period of time. Following this observation, Becker and his associates showed that hyperchylomicronemia occurs at any age following a fat-loaded meal.[22] However, the intensity, size, and duration of the chylomicron state increases with the age of the individual because the clearing mechanisms are lacking or are less active in the older age groups. The abnormal postabsorptive chylomicron state in older human beings may be restored to the normal state by the use of detergents and lipases, such as heparin.[23] These separate observations by Moreton and Becker are interrelated and suggest that a disturbance in the colloidal state of the blood may be one of the most important factors in atherosclerosis. They also support our observation that the absorption and intake of cholesterol is not the only factor involved in atherosclerosis.[24] In addition, they demonstrate the necessity of increasing the rapidity of lipid absorption and utilization in older individuals. These hypotheses were extended by Gofman and later, Fredrickson.

Gofman and his co-workers showed that the blood of individuals with atherosclerosis contained an increased concentration of large cholesterol molecules of the class Sf 10-20. By the implementation of a low-fat, low-cholesterol diet, the concentration of these large molecules was decreased to normal values. On this basis, Gofman recommended the use of a low-cholesterol, low-fat diet. This was upheld by the Inter-Society Commission for Heart Disease Resources.[25] Recent work by Levy, Fredrickson, and their colleagues has extended these observations. Levy and Fredrickson's classification of lipoproteins has clarified to some extent the patterns associated with atheropoiesis and the influence of dietary restrictions on reducing the presence of these lipoproteins in the blood.[26] Thus, it becomes apparent in conformation with Hatch et al. that restriction of carbohydrates, not fat, will reduce lipoprotein pattern type IV, whereas restriction of fats will normalize type II.[27] The observation that type IV hyperlipoproteinemia is influenced by carbohydrate restriction and type II by fat restriction points up the fact that fat and, particularly saturated fat, is not the sole dietary factor in the etiology of atheropoiesis. (See Chapter VI.)

Studies by other investigators

Further support for the dietary causation theory of atherosclerosis is the decrease in atherosclerosis in Germany immediately following World War I.[28] Similar evidence was obtained in the Netherlands and Scandinavia during and shortly after World War II, when the incidence of coronary heart disease paralleled the consumption of total fats and calories.[29] Also cited is the low incidence of atherosclerosis in chronic alcoholics,[30] and the decrease of atherosclerosis in ill-nourished and lean individuals.[31] Critical examination of the data reveals that the authors' claims are based on the assumption that in these groups the fat and cholesterol intake was decreased, thereby decreasing the propensity of the individual to develop atherosclerosis. Actually, ill-nourished individuals and chronic alcoholics are more prone to other diseases at an earlier age and may, therefore, not attain the age at which degenerative diseases manifest themselves. It has been stated that the Chinese population between 1930-1950 did not experience atherosclerosis with the frequency or to the extent that Western civilization did.[32] However, the same author acknowledged that at that time the average life span of the Chinese was 42 years, which is below the age of the development of atherosclerosis in epidemic proportions.

Recent international epidemiological studies have demonstrated that where dietary fats are in excess, coronary heart disease is also in excess. But there are exceptions to these findings. In the developing countries, such as India and Pakistan, coronary heart disease is present in patients whose cholesterol is not elevated and whose dietary fat intake is not excessive by Western standards. The question arises whether the patients observed in developing countries are comparable to patients in the more developed countries in whom coronary heart disease appears despite low cholesterol values and low fat intake. The corollary to this question is whether the incidence of coronary heart disease in these countries will increase when the intake of fat approaches that of the Western countries.

A study conducted on U.S. Marines in basic training at Paris Island revealed a daily dietary intake of 4,500 calories consisting of 45 per cent saturated fats.[33] During this rigorous training of 26 weeks' duration, the serum cholesterol did not vary beyond normal limits. The explanation given was that the saturated fats provided the calories for such energy expenditures. The evidence pointing to ingestion of total fat as being related to atherosclerogenesis stems from epidemiological studies demonstrating that populations whose total caloric intake was less than 15 per cent fat had lower serum cholesterol and less cardiovascular disease than populations whose total diet contained 40 per cent fat.

The evidence from several studies indicates that the levels of serum cholesterol are unrelated to the intake of cholesterol per se. Keys[34] offers this evidence from studies in east and west Finland, where each diet contained 180 mg per 1,000 calories, and serum cholesterol averaged 265 mg per cent and 253 mg per cent for east and west, respectively. In Dalmatia and Montegiorgio, serum cholesterol was 185 mg per cent and 197 mg per cent, respectively, and the intake was 90 mg cholesterol per 1,000 calories. Keys states that virtually no correlation exists between caloric intake and the level of serum cholesterol. This statement is open to considerable discussion because it is based on a population whose caloric intake is much lower than that of the U.S., and where all calories are utilized for activities of daily living. This point is emphasized in the aforementioned study of Marines. At the end of a six-month rigorous training program, the weight change was negligible, as was the serum cholesterol. Thus, it may be inferred that if all calories are expended, regardless of intake, serum cholesterol will be unchanged. Accordingly, it is reasonable to conclude that in those areas where the caloric intake is small, serum cholesterol will probably be low as well, regardless of the dietary cholesterol or fat intake.

The Interrelationships Between Dietary Intake and Blood Coagulation

Although there is no dispute about the association between serum lipids and atheropoiesis, controversy does exist over the exact role serum lipids play in atheropoiesis. Considerable evidence has accumulated during the past decade concerning the relevance of serum lipids to the clotting process. One can hypothesize after reviewing the evidence that even though lipids do accumulate in the arterial walls and compromise the diameter of the vessel, a thrombosis upon the damaged vessel wall may be a secondary effect of the various serum lipids. This hypothesis is not without support.

One of the chief reactions in the clotting process is the conversion of prothrombin to thrombin. This step cannot be accomplished without the enzyme thromboplastin. Thromboplastin is a lipoprotein whose exact composition is not known. However, thromboplastin is thought to be composed of 19 per cent cholesterol, 18 per cent fat, and 63 per cent phospholipids in an alcohol-ether extract. It is generally agreed, however, that in thromboplastin there are at least 15 amino acids and various lipids, such as cholesterol, cerebrosides, gangliosides, and phospholipids. These phospholipids are phosphatidyl derivatives of ethanolamine and sphingomyelin. Phospholipids as a group may act as a substitute for platelet suspensions in the thromboplastin generation test.

The literature contains many excellent papers that document lipids as both procoagulants and anticoagulants. Lipids are classified as phospholipids or fatty acids.

The phospholipids appear to play a common role in coagulation and atherogenesis because they constitute a major portion of thromboplastin, and they are purported to have an inhibitory effect on cholesterol in atherosclerogenesis. Furthermore, it has been well established that the various bases of phospholipids are either pro- or anticoagulant.[35]

Phospholipids are composed of several components, including the following:

a) Lecithin (choline). The crude preparations of lecithin were considered to be clot promoting. However, pure fractions of lecithin are not procoagulant. When lecithin was employed in experiments with Russell's viper venom and in the thromboplastin generation, the results were negative, lending support to the inactivity of pure lecithin.

b) Cephalin (ethanolamine). It is generally agreed that cephalin does not possess a clot promoting property. However, a certain synthetic cephalin—(1 palmitoyl, 3-linoleoyl) 2-phosphatidylethanolamine—does have weak clot promoting properties. According to Rouser, the activity of cephalin rises with the degree of unsaturation of the symmetrically distributed fatty acids of the molecule.[36] It is believed that such compounds do not occur naturally.

c) Phosphatidylserine. Phosphatidylserine prolongs, to a slight degree, the clotting time of plasma, but it shortens the clotting time in Russell's viper venom test. Although the results are contradictory, phosphatidylserine does appear to have some influence on blood clotting.

Despite the inactivity of pure lecithin and cephalin and the weak activity of phosphatidylserine, there is much information concerning the combinations of various phospholipids. The combinations of naturally occurring α structures and L-configuration phospholipids such as choline, cephalin, and serine give support to a coagulation effect. Phosphatidylserine, in combination with phosphatidylethanolamine, produces a clot promoting effect in low concentrations and is inhibitory in higher concentrations. The combinations of PE and PS are similar in action, indicating that it is the production or presence of combinations of negative or positive charges, rather than the phospholipids themselves, that produce the clotting effect.

Blood thromboplastin can be prepared, according to Spaet and Clintron.[37] They noted that a concentration of at least 10 mg of lipid phosphorus per 1 ml of prepared thromboplastin is necessary for activity.

In 1950, Gertler and Garn reported that serum cholesterol rose with age in both controls and C.H.D. subjects.[38] Though there was a concomitant rise in lipid phosphorus in both groups, the rise was much more rapid in the control group than in the C.H.D. group. Accordingly, the protective nature of phospholipids as an anticoagulant may be lost in the proportional decrease of phospholipids.

The Effect of Fatty Acids on Thrombus Formation

The literature is replete with information concerning the effects of fats on the atherogenic process. These have been reviewed in various sections of this monograph. It has been pointed out, however, that certain inconsistencies do occur. For example, studies reveal that individuals from developing countries who have èxperienced myocardial infarctions have serum cholesterol levels in the range of 170-180 mg per cent. Similarly, individuals from relatively developed countries have slightly higher serum cholesterol levels of 200-220 mg per cent. These compare with serum cholesterol levels of approximately 275 mg per cent for patients in the U.S. who have experienced myocardial infarctions.

The common denominator in all these observations is the thrombotic nature of the acute event within the coronary arteries. In an attempt to unify the apparently contradictory observations, a search of the literature was made for data on the effects of various lipids on blood coagulation. Along with studies made in our laboratory, the search yielded information believed to be noteworthy.

Three chief areas of investigation in the literature suggested that fatty acids and phospholipids affect blood coagulation. Connor and Poole demonstrated from in vitro rat blood experiments that thrombus formation varied with the type of fatty acid and the length of the chain.[39] Thus, the long-chain saturated fatty acids from palmitate (^{16}C) to cerotate (^{26}C) resulted in an abbreviated thrombus formation time of 43-59 per cent when compared to a saline control. The intermediate-chain-length saturated fatty acids, such as laurate (^{12}C) and myristate (^{14}C), had some effect in shortening thrombus formation, but the short-chain fatty acids such as caproate (^{6}C) and heptoate (^{7}C) had no effect whatsoever. The long-chain unsaturated fatty acids, that is, oleate (^{18}C) and arachidonate (^{20}C) had no effect on the time of thrombus formation.

The concentration of the fatty acid within wide limits (.001-.07 per cent) did not appear to affect the rate of thrombus formation. Another interesting observation was that when mixtures of unsaturated and saturated acids were tested, the rate of thrombus formation depended on the type of saturated fatty acid present.

There are interesting observations concerning the effects of ethanolamine phosphatide on blood coagulation. Poole and Robinson reported that ethanolamine phosphatide prepared from brain, egg yolk, and organic synthesis shortened the clotting times in the presence of Russell's viper venom and also increased the amount of thrombin generated from plasma.[40] These observations are particularly interesting in view of Dr. Irving Wright's findings that in subjects fed six eggs a day, the prothrombin levels were virtually unchanged. No other coagulation tests were performed by Wright. These findings as well as those to follow were published in the discussion accompanying the article entitled, "The Effect of Ingested Fat on Blood Coagulation," by G. G. Duncan.[41]

Thannhauser observed that in several patients with ideopathic hyperlipemia, whose neutral fats were 20-40 times the normal values, there was no increased tendency to thrombosis. Duncan, on the other hand, states that coagulation time is decreased in hyperlipemic diabetic patients. In a classical study, Duncan observed the effect of ingestion of refined corn oil (unsaturated fats), olive oil (mixed unsaturated and saturated fats), and 40 per cent cream from cow's milk (saturated fats) on the rate of coagulation in dog blood. He concluded that the ingestion of cream, particularly, increases the rate of coagulation both locally and systemically, which may account for the desired effect in gastric or duodenal bleeding. But it obviously causes an undesirable effect on the coronary arteries. Similar though less striking effects were observed with olive oil and corn oil.

Another observation that merits attention is the effect of fatty acids on cardiac metabolism during acute myocardial infarction. Opie as well as Oliver showed that free fatty acids increase as a result of the rise of catecholamine release in acute myocardial infarction. Opie extended these observations and showed that an increase in free fatty acids may produce an uncoupling of oxidative phosphorylation, leading to cardiac dysrhythmias with adverse effects.[42]

A study in which a diet of soybean oil (iodine value 133) and mixed vegetable oils (iodine value 4) was given to two groups of 10 individuals each revealed that changes other than the lowering of serum cholesterol may be the actual beneficial effect of an unsaturated fat diet. For example, in the subjects given soybean oil, platelet factor 3 showed a moderate reduction in activity. In addition, platelet aggregation was decreased in the soybean group and increased in the mixed vegetable oil group.[43]

In another study, there was a definite increase in platelet susceptibility to thrombin-induced aggregation in rats fed butter or stearic acid. These changes did not occur in similar animals fed corn oil, linoleic acid, or oleic acid. These studies were extended to patients with myocardial infarction and men with low risk of coronary heart disease. The observations were similar to those made in the experimental model with rats. Thus, it appears that the thrombotic tendency in experimental rats as well as in men with coronary heart disease was related to platelet aggregation, which was in turn related to the saturated fatty acids in the diet.[44]

In an effort to localize the selective and active area of platelet metabolism as it relates to platelet function, several authors made radioautographic studies employing ^{3}H palmitate and ^{14}C palmitate, coupled with homogenate techniques. The observed site was in the membrane.[45] The physiologic significance of these findings supports observations about the dietary influences of increased adhesiveness and aggregation on platelet metabolism, with a secondary influence on increased tendency to thrombi formation.

Fullerton and his colleagues demonstrated that, saturated or unsaturated, fatty acids as a rule assume various properties relating to thrombosis, depending upon whether they are combined with serum albumins.[46] These authors suggest that saturated fatty acids with 14 carbons have an inhibitory effect on tissue thromboplastins, but that these effects are superseded by the unsaturated fatty acids of ^{16}C chain length. Such studies emphasize the importance of fats in the etiology of ischemic vascular disease.

There is no doubt that fatty acids play an important role in the formation of thrombi. This property is enhanced by the addition of albumin to the experimental mixtures. This observation adds more credence to the concept that lipoproteins contribute much to the etiology of ischemic vascular disease.

Summary

The classical investigations that associate diet with atheropoiesis and, hence, coronary heart disease are based on the following indices: (a) fat ingestion (saturated/unsaturated fat ratios and total amount of fat), (b) cholesterol ingestion, (c) caloric ingestion, and (d) a combination of all three. The conclusions are based on epidemiological studies both in the United States and in many parts of the world. The general conclusions from an empirical standpoint are: (a) Total fat in the diet should not exceed 35 per cent of the total calories, and saturated/unsaturated fat ratio should equal 1:2, and (b) cholesterol intake of under 300 mg per day is considered prudent. These conclusions are not supported by studies our research group made in the Marine Corps, where the average serum cholesterol in the young Marines was virtually unchanged on a daily diet of 4,500 calories consisting of 45 per cent saturated fat. These Marines were on daily maneuvers and utilized these excess calories for heat and energy production. Additional support is derived from our observations in India and Pakistan where the diet is generally low in fat and where serum cholesterol is also low (approximately 160 mg per cent), yet where there is coronary heart disease. Further observations that raise doubts about the fat ingestion and elevated cholesterol theories is the lack of proof that dietary fat is deposited in the arteries.

Sufficient evidence exists for cholesterol and other fatty acid synthesis within the intima and media. Of importance is that carbohydrates in excess may produce fatty acids and, hence, triglycerides, which will find their way into the serum, as in type IV hyperlipoproteinemia. Our own studies revealed higher fat and cholesterol intake in the control group than in the coronary group.

The association between dietary fats and coronary events may be due to other factors in addition to those already cited. A survey of the literature revealed that fats play an important role in blood clotting. Thus, diet may be involved not only in the chronic phase of atheropoiesis but in the acute phase of thrombosis as well. It was pointed out that thromboplastin, an important enzyme that converts prothrombin to thrombin, is composed chiefly of phospholipids. Thus, an alteration of the phospholipids would, theoretically, alter the clotting mechanisms. There has been considerable evidence suggesting that butter or stearic acid favors platelet aggregation. There are other data indicating that short-chain saturated fatty acids favor coagulation, and that long-chain saturated and unsaturated fatty acids inhibit coagulation. Thus, there is no doubt that diet plays a dual role in coronary heart disease; that is, in arterial wall deposition and the coagulation process as well.

References

1 W. Dock, "The Predilection of Atherosclerosis for the Coronary Arteries," *JAMA* 131: 875-878, 1946; I. Snapper, "Nutrition and Nutritional Disease in the Orient," *Adv. Int. Med.* 2: 577-605, 1947.
2 A. Steiner and F. E. Kendall, "Atherosclerosis and Arteriosclerosis in Dogs Following Ingestion of Cholesterol and Thiouracil," *Arch. Path.* 42: 433-444, 1946.
3 B. L. Duff, "Experimental Cholesterol Arteriosclerosis and Its Relationship to Human Arteriosclerosis," *Arch. Path.* 20: 81-123, 259-304, 1935.
4 T. Leary, "Crystalline Ester Cholesterol and Atherosclerosis," *Arch. Path.* 147: 1-28, 1949.
5 Duff, "Experimental Cholesterol."
6 Leary, "Crystalline Ester," pp. 1-28.
7 R. Schoenheimer and F. Breusch, "Synthesis and Destruction of Cholesterol in the Organism," *J. Biol. Chem.* 103: 439-448, 1933; K. Bloch, "Biological Synthesis of Cholesterol," *Harvey Lectures* 48: 68-88, 1952; F. Lynen, H. Eggerer, U. Henning, and I. Kessel, "Farnesyl-Pyrophosphat und 3-Methyl-Δ^3-Butenyl-1-Pyrophosphat, die Biologischen Varstufen der Squalens," *Angew. Chem.* 70: 738, 1958; J. D. Brodie, G. Wasson, and J. W. Porter, "The Participation of Malonyl Coenzyme in the Biosynthesis of Mevalonic Acid," *J. Biol. Chem.* 238: 1294-1301, 1963.
8 A. Ladd, A. Kellner, and J. W. Correll, "Intravenous Detergents in Experimental Atherosclerosis With Special Reference to the Possible Role of Phospholipids," *Fed. Proc.* Part I, 8: 360, 1949.
9 S. L. Wilens, "The Relationship of Chronic Alcoholism to Atherosclerosis," *JAMA* 135: 1136-1139, 1947.
10 L. Aschoff, *Lectures in Pathology* (New York: P. B. Hoeber, 1924), pp. 131-153; A. Keys, Personal communication.
11 W. J. Walker, "Relationship of Adiposity to Serum Cholesterol and Lipoprotein Levels and Their Modification by Dietary Means," *Ann. Int. Med.* 39: 705-716, 1953.
12 J. Stamler, *Lectures on Preventive Cardiology* (New York: Grune and Stratton, 1967), p. 187; H. Blackburn and J. Willis, eds., "The Minnesota Symposium on Prevention in Cardiology–Reducing the Risk of Coronary and Hypertensive Disease," *Minn. Med.* 52(8), 1969.
13 H. B. Lofland, R. W. St. Clair, T. B. Clarkson et al., "Atherosclerosis in Cebus Monkeys. II. Arterial Metabolism," *Exp. Molec. Path.* 9: 57, 1968.
14 R. W. St. Clair, H. B. Lofland, R. W. Prichard et al., "Synthesis of Squalene and Sterols by Isolated Segments of Human and Pigeon Arteries," *Exp. Molec. Path.* 8: 201, 1968.
15 A. J. Day, H. A. Newman, and D. B. Zilversmit, "Synthesis of Phospholipid by Foam Cells Isolated From Rabbit Atherosclerotic Lesions," *Circ. Res.* 19: 22, 1966; H. A. Newman, E. L. McCandless, and D. B. Zilversmit, "The Synthesis of C^{14} Lipids in Rabbit Atheromatous Lesions," *J. Biol. Chem.* 236: 1264, 1961.
16 M. W. Bitts and D. Kritchevsky, "Observations With Radioactive Hydrogen (H^3) in Experimental Atherosclerosis," *Circulation* 4: 34, 1961.
17 H. P. Dustan, "Atherosclerosis Complicating Chronic Hypertension," *Circulation* 50: 871-879, 1974.
18 C. Kang-Jey Ho, B. Taylor, and K. Biss, "Overall Control of Sterol Synthesis in Animals and Man," in *Atherosclerosis: Proceedings of the Second International Symposium on Atherosclerosis* (New York: Springer-Verlag, 1970) pp. 271-273.
19 D. S. Goodman, "The Measurement of Cholesterol Pools and Turnover in Man," in *Atherosclerosis: Proceedings of the Second International Symposium on Atherosclerosis* (New York: Springer-Verlag, 1970). pp. 242-248.
20 J. R. Moreton, "Physical State of Lipids, and Foreign Substances Producing Atherosclerosis," *Science* 107: 371-373, 1948.
21 J. W. Gofman, F. T. Lindgren, H. A. Elliot et al., "The Role of Lipids and Lipoproteins in Atherosclerosis," *Science* 111: 166-171, 1950.
22 G. H. Becker, J. Meyer, and H. Necheles, "Fat Absorption and Atherosclerosis," *Science* 110:529-530, 1949.
23 C. B. Anfinsen, E. Boyle, and R. K. Brown, "The Role of Heparin in Lipoprotein Metabolism," *Science* 115: 583-586, 1952.
24 M. M. Gertler and S. M. Garn, "The Lipid Interrelationship in Health and in Coronary Artery Disease," *Science* 112: 14-16, 1950.
25 "Report of Inter-Society Commission for Heart Disease Resources: Primary Prevention of the Atherosclerotic Diseases," *Circulation* 42: A55-95, 1970.
26 R. I. Levy and D. S. Fredrickson, "Diagnosis and Management of Hyperlipoproteinemia," *Am. J. Cardiol.* 22(4): 576-583, 1968.
27 F. T. Hatch, L. L. Abell, and F. E. Kendall, "Effects of Restriction of Dietary Fat and Cholesterol Upon Serum Lipids and Lipoproteins in Patients With Hypertension," *Amer. J. Med.* 19: 48, 1955.
28 Aschoff, *Lectures in Pathology.*
29 I. Vartiainen and K. Kanerva, "Arterio-

sclerosis and Wartime," *Ann. Med. Int. Fenn.* 36: 748, 1947.
30 Wilens, "Relationship of Chronic Alcoholism," pp. 1136-1139.
31 S. L. Wilens, "The Bearing of the General Nutritional State on Atherosclerosis," *Arch. Int. Med.* 79: 129-147, 1947.
32 L. Snapper, *Chinese Lessons to Western Medicine,* 1st ed. (New York: Interscience Publishers, Inc., 1941), p. 380.
33 G. L. Calvy, L. D. Cady, M. X. Mufson et al., "Serum Lipids and Enzymes," *JAMA* 183: 1-4, 1963.
34 A. Keys, ed., "Coronary Heart Disease in Seven Countries," *Circulation* 51 (Suppl. 1): 1-211, 1970.
35 M. M. Gertler, J. Kream, and O. Baturay, "Studies on the Phosphatide Content of Human Serum," *J. Biol. Chem.* 207: 165-173, 1954; E. Chargaff, C. Levine, C. Green, "Techniques for the Demonstration by Chromatography of Nitrogenous Lipide Constituents, Sulphur-Containing Amino Acids, and Reducing Sugars," *J. Biol. Chem.* 75: 67-71, 1948; E. Hecht and H. Ottens, "Die Bedeutung der Lipoide fur Blutgerinnung. 1. Mitt. Den Einfluss der Monoaminophosphatide (Insbes. des Lecithins) und Einger Anderer Lipoide, Einschliesslich deren Spaltungsprodukte," *Acta Haemat. (Basel)* 8: 265-276, 1952.
36 G. Rouser and D. Schloredt, "Phospholipid Structure and Thromboplastic Activity II. The Fatty Acid Composition of the Active Phosphatidyl Ethanolamine," *Biochem. Biophys. Acta.* 28: 81-86, 1958.
37 T. H. Spaet and J. Clintron, "Blood Thromboplastin: Its Preparation and Properties," *Proc. Soc. Exp. Biol. Med.* 101: 799-801, 1959.
38 M. M. Gertler and S. M. Garn, "The Interrelationships of Serum Cholesterol, Cholesterol Esters, and Phospholipids in Health and in Coronary Artery Disease," *Circulation* II (2): 205-214, 1950.
39 W. E. Connor and J. C. F. Poole, "The Effect of Fatty Acids on the Formation of Thrombi," *Quart. J. Exp. Physiol.* 46(1): 1-7, 1961.
40 J. C. F. Poole and D. S. Robinson, "Further Observations on the Effects of Ethanolamine Phosphatide on Plasma Coagulation," *Quart. J. Exp. Physiol.* 41(3): 295-300, 1956.
41 G. G. Duncan and J. M. Waldron, "The Effect of Ingested Fat on Blood Coagulation," *Tr. A. Am. Phys.* 62: 179-185, 1940.
42 L. H. Opie, "Metabolic Response During Impending Myocardial Infarction. 1. Relevance of Studies of Glucose and Fatty Acid Metabolism in Animals," *Circulation* 45: 483-490, 1972; M. F. Oliver, "Metabolic Response During Impending Myocardial Infarction. II. Clinical Implications," *Circulation* 45: 491-500, 1972.
43 A. Nordoy and J. M. Rodset, "The Influence of Dietary Fats on Platelets in Man," *Acta Med. Scand.* 190: 27-34, 1971.
44 S. Renaud, K. Kuba, C. Gonlet et al., "Relationship Between Fatty-Acid Composition of Platelets and Platelet Aggregation in Rat and Man," *Circulation Research* 26: 553-564, 1970.
45 J. C. Hoak, A. A. Spector, G. L. Fry et al., "Localization of Free Fatty Acids Taken Up by Human Platelets," *Blood* 40(1): 16-22, 1972.
46 W. W. Fullerton, W. A. Boggust, and R. A. Q. O'Meara, "Antithromboplastic and Thromboplastic Activities of Free Fatty Acids," *J. Clin. Path.* 20: 624-628, 1967.

IX Coagulation Factors

The risk factor concept in coronary heart disease has made it possible to single out individuals who are particularly prone to the disease.

Since 1966, our laboratory has advanced the theory that it should be possible to determine not only *who* the candidate for coronary heart disease is but also *when* the event will take place.

There is little argument that what pushes covert coronary heart disease into its acute, overt, symptomatic stage is a compromising of the coronary artery, which curtails adequate blood flow commensurate with myocardial demand. There is a preponderance of evidence to suggest that the compromise is due to thrombotic events superimposed on an atherosclerotic process.[1] This investigation team has evidence that the final thrombotic event is a gradual process that can be spotted by systematic serial examination of the blood coagulation process. When the blood coagulation profile shows a predominance of procoagulants, due either to an increase in procoagulants or a decrease in natural anticoagulants or inhibitors, then the blood may be termed hypercoagulable. Our hypothesis is that the final series of events that compromises the coronary lumen in C.H.D. is a change in coagulation factors, in which the procoagulants dominate the anticoagulant and fibrinolytic systems, resulting in fibrin formation. There is sufficient evidence to show that periodic examinations of coagulation parameters will detect a change in the state of coagulability.

The Coagulation Mechanisms

Texon and other investigators accumulated substantial data from animal studies and autopsy reports showing that the atherosclerotic process has a predilection for those areas of the arteries that are subject to shearing and drag forces and changes in the pressure gradients, all of which cause stretching and contraction of vessel walls.[2] These investigators also emphasized that focal lesions are present in areas where there are curves, anastomoses, and narrowings. Duguid extended these findings by applying basic physiology and biochemistry to his histologic observations. He firmly believed in Rokitansky's theory that atheromas are caused by thrombi adhering to the vessel wall,[3] and demonstrated that fibrin deposits are the result of naturally occurring substances, such as platelets, rather than degenerative processes, as claimed by Virchow.[4] The proponents of this theory maintain that the fibrinogen-thromboplastic system can be favorable or unfavorable to these deposits and either allow the clot to remain or destroy it, depending on the ability of the fibrinolysins to dissolve the fibrin.

The theories of Virchow, Rokitansky, Duguid, and others have a common denominator. Their apparent differences lie only in the emphasis each author gives to his own viewpoint. Each of their observations is correct, but each refers to a different pathologic-physiologic sequence in the atherosclerotic process. Thus, Virchow's recognition of and emphasis on degeneration is correct, though degeneration is only one phase of the atherosclerotic process. Rokitansky's and Duguid's observations and interpretations are also correct, insofar as they represent another phase of the atherosclerotic process. The modern concept of coagulation-thrombosis-fibrinolysis has been closely associated with the lipid theory ever since it was established that lipids tend to produce arterial degeneration as well as influence blood clotting (see Chapter VIII).

The blood clotting process can be outlined in three stages involving 13 factors. Each stage has a special function; together they form a continuum. From a biochemical viewpoint, the blood clotting process is a series of coupled reactions that result in fibrin formation. The reactions are not all known or understood, but progress is currently being made toward that end together with advances in biochemistry and biophysics.

Stage I reactions essentially involve the activation of a series of proteins in a sequential (or cascading) manner. This action is completed when thromboplastin is formed. The conversion of prothrombin to thrombin in stage II is virtually impossible without the aid of thromboplastin. Thromboplastin may be derived from both an intrinsic (contact-activated) and extrinsic (tissue-activated) system. These two systems have some similarities and some differences. The intrinsic system involves factors VIII, IX, XI, and XII; the extrinsic system involves factor VII and the tissue factor. The factors that both systems share are factors II, V, X, as well as phospholipid and calcium.

Thrombin is a powerful esterase and protease that converts fibrinogen into fibrin. It is virtually nonexistent in the blood, but is derived from prothrombin at an enormous rate when the conversion reaction begins. Prothrombin has a half-life of 3-4 days. The factors involved in stage II are factors II, IV, V, X, X_a, phospholipid, and calcium. Factor X may be activated to factor X_a (or thrombokinase) by extrinsic factors with factor VII and by intrinsic factors VIII, IX, and XII, or by Russell's viper venom. These sequences have been challenged somewhat by Seegers, but it appears that these differences are not ones of substance but rather of semantics.[5] Thrombin also activates factors V, VIII, and XIII (fibrin stabilizing factor).

In simple terms, thrombin hydrolyzes the arginyl-glycine bond as well as other bonds in fibrinogen, converting it into fibrin, the stable and visible end product of the clotting process in stage III. This happens if the thrombin fails to be neutralized by the antithrombins (particularly antithrombin III). Failure on the part of this damping system will result in clot formation. Additional homeostatic mechanisms come into action to obviate the final phase of clot formation. Two of the most notable mechanisms are the formation of antithrombin VI from the action of the plasminogen system and euglobulin.

By assaying these enzyme systems and the level of fibrinogen itself, one can assess the degree of clot formation and the homeostatic protective devices that become operative during the coagulation crisis. It is reasonable to assume that such a complex biochemical mechanism would have to have counter processes to maintain homeostasis and keep a check on the forces promoting clot formation. If this were not so, the blood would become a solid mass.

Design and Background of Our Studies

Our studies on the time at which the biochemical reactions favoring coagulation in the coronary arteries occurs are based on the theory that clot formation progresses in a methodical, predictable manner. Accordingly, tests were devised to determine the integrity of each of the three phases of the clotting mechanism as well as the natural inhibitors. It would have been impossible to study all the factors, so only those we thought could best define the mechanisms of the various phases were chosen.

Stage I
Kaolin-activated partial thromboplastin time
(cephalin clotting time)

This stage I reaction is an improvement of the partial thromboplastin and recalcification times. It is an over-all test of the integrity and clotting ability of stage I in that it indicates the physiologic functional levels of factors I, II, V, VIII, IX, X, XI, and XII. Thus, if the reaction is shortened, it indicates an excessive production of activated thromboplastin; conversely, if the reaction is prolonged, it indicates a reduced amount of one or more of the factors. The test has its disadvantages, but it is still an excellent over-all indicator of the integrity of stage I in the clotting scheme.

Stage II
Thrombin activity

Thrombin, as such, does not exist in whole blood in detectable amounts. But its precursor, prothrombin, does. Thus, if the conversion of prothrombin to thrombin is complete, the thrombin can be assayed in an isolated system. The system used in this laboratory measures the acid derived from p-toluenesulfonyl-L-arginine methyl ester (TAME) by the cleavage of thrombin (esterase fraction), which has the advantage of being free from antithrombin effect. The amount of free thrombin available is important because the most rapid chemical reaction in clot formation is the action of thrombin on fibrinogen. An unopposed elevation or presence of thrombin is very important in clot formation.

Stage III

The levels of plasma fibrinogen were studied as an indicator of continuous clot formation. The availability of fibrinogen appeared to be related to blood coagulability.

Inhibitors of coagulation

At the beginning of this chapter it was stated that, in addition to the factors responsible for clot formation, there are other factors that constantly keep the coagulation process from going forward at an undesirable rate, or inhibitors of coagulation.

The inhibitors chosen for study were those involved with thrombosis, namely, antithrombin III, and those concerned with the destruction of the clot itself, the fibrinolysins. These two elements were of particular interest to us since they represented the most important variables in the coagulation process. The enzyme thrombin is what converts the preclotting material (fibrinogen) into a clot (fibrin). An inhibitor of thrombin would prevent the clotting reaction from occurring. In the event that a clot did occur, its inhibitors and solvents could prevent damage resulting from the blockage of the vital coronary or cerebral vessels by rapidly removing the clot.

Antithrombin III

Six types of antithrombins have been described. Antithrombin III is a protein that destroys or inactivates thrombin with a second-order reaction or through irreversible inhibition. In a clinical or special situation where there is an accelerated production of clotting enzymes, which is feasible when the kaolin-activated P.T.T. is shortened, homeostatic mechanisms spur greater antithrombin III production.

Antithrombin III production is useful for other biologic reactions. Egberg has suggested that a deficiency in antithrombin III produces a tendency toward thrombosis.[6] While this is a reasonable assumption, there has been evidence opposing this view. This laboratory has developed a method for measuring antithrombin III.[7] It is based on the rivanol inactivation of α_2 macroglobulin without affecting the activity of antithrombin III. This measurement, in conjunction with other measurements, plays an important role in our linear regression formula for assessing the coagulation propensity of blood.

Fibrinolytic system

For some time it had been known that the blood from animals killed after a long and hard chase did not readily clot. But the factors responsible for this phenomenon were not understood until Tillet and Garner established that the culture medium of certain strains of hemolytic streptococci contained a substance that could lyse human blood clots.[8] When it was added to the euglobulin fraction of human serum, purified human fibrin, it was found, could be lysed.[9] Soon it was established that there were four parts to this (fibrinolytic or plasminogen-plasma) system: plasminogen, plasmin, activators, and inhibitors. The activation of plasminogen into plasmin is achieved mainly through the use of urokinase, but other proteolytic enzymes such as trypsin and its product plasmin may be involved, as well as streptokinase, and lysokinase. Following a myocardial infarction, tissue activators of plasminogen are seen in the connective tissue. The activator urokinase also appears in the urine in increased quantities during acute myocardial infarction.

In biological terms, the fibrinolytic system is the last defense against the harmful effects of a clot. So measuring fibrinolytic activity together with fibrinogen levels will indicate the rapidity with which fibrinogen is being removed or converted. It may also suggest the degree to which this is due to increased fibrinolytic activity, which may be judged by the fact that the half-life of fibrinogen is 4-6 days and that a minimum of 50-100 mg/100 ml plasma is required for homeostasis.[10] Thus, if the fibrinogen levels fall faster than the estimated half-life, it will be a good indication of rapid utilization in the presence of increased fibrinolytic activity.

Results of Coagulation Studies

Blood coagulation studies were performed on the original control group, although logistical problems made it difficult to perform the coagulation tests generally performed in this laboratory. Subjects were divided into two groups, according to our linear regression formula, to determine high and low risk for C.H.D.[11] Table 9.1 summarizes the coagulation findings of these two groups.

The statistical evaluation revealed that the high-risk group had a significantly lower kaolin-activated P.T.T. level than the low-risk group. Thus, the high-risk individuals had a more procoagulant status. There were no significant differences observed between the two groups in plasminogen or prothrombin levels.

Further follow-up studies of this group will be required to verify our hypothesis. Since these studies were performed, additional coagulation parameters have been added to our investigations. More complete data are available for another series investigated by this group. They are reported herein.

Coagulation studies were performed on various groups of coronary heart disease patients, as well as on groups of healthy individuals who had been classified into high- and low-risk categories for C.H.D. Table 9.2 shows that (a) the lowest prothrombin level occurred in the acute M.I. group, and the highest in the healthy high-risk group; (b) the K.P.T.T. was lowest in the acute M.I. group and highest in the chronic M.I. group treated with minidose heparin; (c) the fibrinogen levels were not significantly different; thus, highest and lowest levels were meaningless in the groups studied; (d) antithrombin III levels were lowest in the low-risk group and highest in the M.I. group; (e) E.L.T. (euglobulin lysis time) values were lowest in the low-risk group and highest in the acute M.I. group; and (f) plasminogen activity was equally low in the low- and high-risk groups and highest in the acute M.I. group.

The data were analyzed for significant differences among the various groups (Table 9.3). The greatest number of differences (six) appeared in the antithrombin III parameter; four occurred in the K.P.T.T. and prothrombin categories; and there was only one significant difference in the areas of E.L.T. and plasminogen. Fibrinogen levels were not significantly different.

The analysis of the differences in the means gives some insight into the significance of these parameters. It appears that antithrombin III is the most important parameter in determining the differences in blood coagulability. The K.P.T.T., by virtue of having the greatest degree of difference, is second in importance and prothrombin levels, third.

These differences suggest that a mechanistic approach to the evaluation of blood coagulability in the various groups is possible. It appears that there are at least several mechanisms that occur simultaneously. Antithrombin III serves as a protective mechanism, rising only when necessary to neutralize thrombin during acute M.I. or in high-risk cases where the activation of thrombin occurs more rapidly, as evidenced by low K.P.T.T.

Table 9.1 1971 coagulation results for control group based on profile score

Category	Number	Profile score Mean ± S.D.	K.P.T.T. Mean ± S.D.	Prothrombin Mean ± S.D.	Plasminogen Mean ± S.D.
Low-risk	12	36.3 ± 12.95	39.7 ± 6.75	50.1 ± 7.0	1.30 ± 0.32
High-risk	8	80.9 ± 15.65	34.6 ± 3.23	52.1 ± 9.54	1.38 ± 0.17

Table 9.2 Mean values of coagulation parameters in healthy low-risk, high-risk, chronic, and acute M.I. groups*

			Prothrombin	K.P.T.T.	Fibrinogen	Anti III	E.L.T.	Plasminogen
Group	Age	Number	Mean ± S.D.	Mean ± S.D.	Mean ± S.D.	Mean ± S.D.	Mean ± S.D.	Mean ± S.D.
Healthy low-risk	51	33	46.0 ± 9.51	41.5 ± 5.07	381 ± 74.3	516 ± 58	309 ± 66	1.37 ± 0.25
Healthy high-risk	50	31	51.6 ± 8.97	40.5 ± 6.62	374 ± 63.9	564 ± 58.6	346 ± 84.2	1.37 ± 0.22
Chronic M.I. (no drugs)	54	34	47.1 ± 8.99	42.2 ± 5.23	372 ± 74.5	551 ± 58	340 ± 67.5	1.26 ± 0.29
Chronic M.I. (heparin)	53	13	–	42.7 ± 6.39	367 ± 85.6	532 ± 40	–	–
Acute M.I.	53	14	41.5 ± 8.25	30.9 ± 3.25	387 ± 116	640 ± 71	352 ± 64.6	1.48 ± 0.29

*Based on profile score below 33 for low-risk and above 62.2 for high-risk patients.

Table 9.3 T-tests for significant differences in coagulation parameters between healthy low-risk, high-risk, chronic, and acute M.I. groups

Group Comparison	Prothrombin	K.P.T.T.	Fibrinogen	Anti III	E.L.T.	Plasminogen
Low-risk/high-risk	.05	ns	ns	.01	ns	ns
Low-risk/chronic M.I. (no drugs)	ns	ns	ns	.05	ns	ns
Low-risk/chronic M.I. (heparin)	–	ns	ns	ns	–	–
Low-risk/acute M.I.	.05	.001	ns	.001	.05	ns
High-risk/chronic M.I. (no drugs)	ns	ns	ns	ns	ns	ns
High-risk/chronic M.I. (heparin)	–	ns	ns	ns	–	–
High-risk/acute M.I.	.001	.001	ns	.001	ns	ns
Chronic M.I./chronic M.I. (no drugs) (heparin)	–	ns	ns	ns	–	–
Chronic M.I./acute M.I. (no drugs)	.05	.001	ns	.001	ns	.05
Chronic M.I./acute M.I. (heparin)	–	.001	ns	.001	–	–

This hypothesis is supported by the observation that E.L.T. displays significant differences where there is virtually no requirement for this mechanism—that is, in low-risk subjects—and where there is a great need for this mechanism, as in acute M.I. patients.

Thus, frequent measurements of these parameters could, over a long period, lead to an indication of increased coagulability. This hypothesis led to the development of a linear regression formula for determining hypercoagulability in high-risk individuals.

The discriminant function

The six coagulation variables used in developing the discriminant function were kaolin-activated partial thromboplastin time, antithrombin III, plasminogen, euglobulin lysis time, fibrinogen, and prothrombin. The linear discriminant function entered the variables in a stepwise manner; thus, at each step of the analysis, variables not yet entered into the function were tested to select the most discriminating variable. In addition, the F ratio was calculated and tested to ensure that each risk factor contributed significantly to the discrimination between healthy age-matched controls and those with an impending acute event.

Two of the six variables proved to be significant discriminators, and the following function for a coagulation profile was determined:

Coagulability score: $-0.326 \times (\text{K.P.T.T.}) + 0.021 \times (\text{Anti III}) + 0.128$

Using only these two factors, the profile misclassified three males in the control group. Eighty-seven per cent of all subjects were identified correctly. The order of the remaining coagulation parameters in discriminating ability was: plasminogen, euglobulin lysis time, fibrinogen, and prothrombin. None of these variables had significant discriminating power. A coagulation profile score above zero identified the individual approaching the acute event, whereas a score below zero identified those subjects exhibiting a normal or eucoagulable state.

Examples of coagulation profile scores for a healthy male and a male who later developed myocardial infarction are given below:

Healthy		Impending acute coronary event	
Antithrombin III	= 469	Antithrombin III	= 689
Kaolin P.T.T.	= 43.2	Kaolin P.T.T.	= 32.0
Coagulability score	= –3.95	Coagulability score	= +4.10

Further insight into the accumulated coagulation data was gained by studying the correlation coefficients, of which the significant ones are summarized in Table 9.4. The positive correlation between antithrombin III and coronary heart disease profile score indicates that increased coagulability takes place as the profile score becomes greater, reflecting increased susceptibility to heart disease. The negative correlation between K.P.T.T. and age suggests that as an individual grows older, there is an increased propensity towards coagulation. Thus, both age and profile score can be indicators of an increased propensity towards coagulation difficulties. The relationship between antithrombin III and K.P.T.T. is strengthened by the strong negative correlation between them. Thus, as K.P.T.T. decreases (an indication of procoagulation), antithrombin III necessarily increases to maintain homeostasis.

Table 9.4 Significant coefficients of correlation for total study population between coagulation and clinical and biochemical variables

Correlations	r	p<
Fibrinogen–sed. rate	.5719	.001
E.L.T.–sed. rate	.2716	.01
Antithrombin III–heart profile score	.2486	.01
Prothrombin–heart profile score	.2082	.05
Antithrombin III–K.P.T.T.	–.2624	.001
Plasminogen–K.P.T.T.	–.2089	.05
Fibrinogen–E.L.T.	–.2107	.01
K.P.T.T.–age	–.1793	.05
Prothrombin–fibrinogen	–.2086	.05
Fibrinogen–systolic B.P.	.1875	.05
E.L.T.–cholesterol	–.1711	.05

The Action of Anticoagulant Drugs

The foregoing appraisal of the various clotting factors represents only the start of a new era in the study of C.H.D. In the future we should be able to anticipate the acute event by recognizing the change that takes place in the blood clotting process, in which the clotting factors shift from a homeostatic to a procoagulative state. If such change is recognized, interference could be applied to the various blood factors to either nullify their action or restore their balance towards the normal range.

The purpose of this chapter is not to discuss the merits of anticoagulation in the prevention of acute overt thrombotic events, either coronary or cerebral. Still, it is worth noting that virtually all of the anticoagulants employed were oral and of the coumadin, dicumarol, or indanedione series. These drugs interfere with the production of prothrombin, but they have no direct effect on thrombin or stage III.

An important but rarely discussed quality of these drugs is their effect on oxidative phosphorylation. Dicumarol uncouples oxidative phosphorylation and, hence, may be somewhat harmful or contraindicated in situations where maximal oxidative phosphorylation is required (for example, in coronary heart disease or ischemic thrombotic cerebrovascular disease where tissue is already oxygen-deprived from curtailed blood supply).

Anticoagulation therapy must be carried out with a knowledge of the total coagulation picture and then applied to the specific areas where interference is desired. In fact, more than one anticoagulant may be required. The following paragraphs outline the principles involved, but their application must be determined by the individual case.

Stage I interference

When K.P.T.T. is shortened in the absence of acute injury, therapy is directed against the formation of thromboplastin by interfering with the intrinsic system. Primary interference with platelet aggregation is achieved by administering an ADP (adenosine diphosphate) inhibitor, such as Persantine (dipyridamole) or aspirin (acetylsalicylic acid), in the second phase.[12] Drugs such as phenylbutazone (Butazolidin) and indomethacin

(Indocin) interfere with platelet adhesiveness. Clofibrate (Atromid-S), an antilipemic agent, also interferes with platelet adhesiveness, but its effect may be an indirect one through its action on the lipids (see Chapter VI). The following agents act on the first and second stages of platelet aggregation and adhesiveness: first stage—dipyridamole, glyceryl trinitrate, guanidine succinic acid (which is present in uremia), and phenylbutazone; second stage—aspirin, phenothiazide, prostaglandin E; platelet adhesiveness—clofibrate, ethylestrenol, phenformin, and saturated fats.

Stage II interference

Interfering with the procoagulant factors in stage II depends on (a) decreasing the amount of prothrombin synthesis, (b) preventing synthesis of factors VII, IX, X, and (c) directly inhibiting thrombin formation. Steps a and b are treated best with coumadin, dicumarol, or the indanedione drugs. These fall short, however, because they do not completely stop synthesis of the factors mentioned. This is illustrated by the direct measurement of the half-life (T 1/2) of various factors, for example, T 1/2=6 hours for factor VII and T 1/2=60 hours for prothrombin. These drugs also have no effect on thrombin itself. Thus the main purpose of the anticoagulation regimen is less than optimally served.

Heparin is probably the best anticoagulant for stage II because it (a) prevents the prothrombin-to-thrombin reaction, (b) inhibits the thrombin-fibrinogen reaction, (c) combines with (along with its cofactor α_2 globulin or antithrombin III) and inactivates thrombin, (d) inhibits (along with its cofactor) factor X_a, which prevents the conversion of prothrombin to thrombin, and (e) activates a plasma lipase that has a clearing property and may affect the entire clotting process.[13]

Thus there are choices of oral anticoagulants for stage II, including dicumarol, indanedione, and the parenterally administered drug, heparin.

Stage III interference

Stage III anticoagulant drugs are concerned with the prevention of fibrin formation and the removal of already formed fibrin.

It is now quite apparent that fibrin formation can be prevented by subverting the fibrinogen-to-fibrin reaction. In the event this fails, however, one can destroy the fibrinogen. The purified venom from the Malayan pit viper (Ancistrodon rhodostoma), commercially called Ancrod or Arvin, contains a property that produces six acidic peptides of fibrin that are removed rapidly from the circulation. Ancrod destroys fibrinogen by breaking it into smaller unstable monomers of fibrin, thus preventing clot formation.

Since fibrinogen is the precursor of fibrin, an important constituent of both thrombosis and clotting, it would seem reasonable to reduce the level of fibrinogen below homeostatic levels, or to 50-100 mg/100 ml plasma, during acute periods to prevent further thrombosis or clotting. Such studies are in progress.

Case History

A healthy male, age 57, came to the clinic on Oct. 13, 1972, because his brother had died of "a heart attack" three months earlier at age 50. His coagulation profile was as follows:

	K.P.T.T.	Antithrombin III	Fibrinogen
10/13/72	44.6	479	325
5/1/73	38.3	518	291
9/25/73*	43.3	581	361
12/5/73	37.4	701	550
12/13/73	37.0	666	514
12/20/73	35.3	662	543

*(The patient took aspirin for a cold several days prior to coming to clinic.)

The patient was periodically followed and K.P.T.T., antithrombin III, and fibrinogen remained stable. The patient was symptom-free. On Dec. 1, 1973, the patient experienced "indigestion" and pain in the precordium, but ignored the symptoms. He later came in on December 5, after calling to relate his symptoms. Blood samples drawn that day revealed normal S.G.O.T. (serum glutamate-oxalacetic transaminase), normal CPK (creatine phosphokinase), and normal resting ECG. The blood coagulation picture revealed a decreased K.P.T.T., and a rise in antithrombin III and fibrinogen. These changes persisted on Dec. 12 and Dec. 20. The ECG, which began to reveal an evolving posterior M.I. on Dec. 13, stabilized by Dec. 20. The patient was symptom-free, and no enzyme changes were detected. The interpretation was that the patient had experienced a "silent M.I." when he developed a hypercoagulable state around Dec. 1.

This case illustrates that a decrease in K.P.T.T. and an increase in antithrombin III precedes the acute overt episode of myocardial infarction. There are 27 other cases with similar histories presently in our records.

Summary

Atheropoiesis may be divided into two stages: (a) lipid deposition or synthesis within the intima and media and (b) changes in the homeostatic mechanisms of coagulation, including the progression from platelet deposition to fibrin production and, hence, thrombosis and compromise of the arterial lumen. Certain physical qualities in the coronary arteries themselves may contribute to the over-all process. These include shearing or drag forces and changes in pressure gradients, which cause the arteries to expand and retract.

Blood clotting appears to consist of a continuous interplay between procoagulant and anticoagulant forces. When the blood coagulation profile indicates a predominance of procoagulants, due either to an increase in procoagulants or a decrease in natural anticoagulants or inhibitors, the blood may be referred to as being in a hypercoagulable state. To back up this theory, measurements were taken at each of the three clotting phases for both the procoagulant and anticoagulant factors in many members of the original control group (classified by high- and low-risk criteria), in a group of acute myocardial infarction patients, and in a group of chronic C.H.D. patients.

The two coagulation parameters that revealed the most interesting results were kaolin-activated partial thromboplastin time and antithrombin III. In the original control group, subjects considered to be high-risk had a lower K.P.T.T. than those who were low-risk. A similar trend was noted in the acute M.I. group when they were compared with low- and high-risk C.H.D. subjects as well as chronic C.H.D. subjects (values of 30.9 versus 41.5). In contrast, antithrombin III levels were significantly elevated (values over 600) in acute M.I. subjects compared to low- and high-risk C.H.D. subjects as well as chronic C.H.D. patients (values from 516 to 564).

These data point to the new concept of hypercoagulability: One can determine by serial, long-term evaluations of coagulation variables whether a subject is experiencing a gradual increase towards hypercoagulability. The case history presented in this chapter supports this contention. Thus, as the K.P.T.T. decreases and antithrombin III increases, concomitantly, an individual approaches or enters into a state of hypercoagulability. One may infer that there is a gradual transition from the covert stage of coronary heart disease to the overt state of the disease via hypercoagulability. It may be possible to prevent this transition by instituting individualized preventive therapy to delay or ameliorate the acute or overt event. It is likely that additional coagulation variables, such as platelet aggregation and heparin levels, will be added to the coagulation profile in the future.

Another area of investigation, which is now in its infancy, is the biological significance of platelet factor IV. This factor has antiheparin properties and thus permits platelets to adhere and aggregate without the interference of heparin on thrombin which helps to enhance these platelet reactions. Platelet factor IV, which is now included in the measurement of heparin neutralizing activity (HNA), has been demonstrated to be elevated in acute myocardial infarction.[14]

References

1 S. Wessler, "The Role of Hypercoagulability in Venous and Arterial Thrombosis," *Cardiovasc. Clin.* 3: 1-16, 1971.

2 M. Texon, "The Role of Vascular Dynamics in the Development of Atherosclerosis," in *Atherosclerosis and Its Origins*, M. Sandler and G. H. Bourne, eds. (New York: Academic Press, 1963) pp. 167-195; G. C. Willis, "Localizing Factors in Atherosclerosis," *Canad. Med. Ass. J.* 70: 1-8, 1954; C. H. Schwartz and R. A. Mitchell, "Observations on Localization of Arterial Plaques," *Circ. Res.* 11: 63-73, 1962.

3 C. Rokitansky, *A Manual of Pathological Anatomy*, vol. 4, trans. G. E. Day, (Philadelphia: Blanchard and Lea, 1855), pp. 1-375.

4 J. B. Duguid, "Pathogenesis of Arteriosclerosis," *Lancet* 2: 925-927, 1949; J. B. Duguid, "Mural Thrombosis in Arteries," *Brit. Med. Bull.* 2: 36-38, 1955; R. Virchow, "Phlogose und Thrombose im Gefassystem," in *Gesammelte Abhandlungen zur Wissenschnftlechen Medicine* (Frankfurt-am-Main: Meidinger Sohn and Co., 1856), p. 458.

5 W. H. Seegers, "Blood Clotting Mechanisms. Three Basic Reactions," *Annual Review of Physiology* 31: 269-294, 1933.

6 O. Egberg, "Inherited Antithrombin Deficiency Causing Thrombophilia," *Thrombosis et Diathesis Haemorrhagica* 13: 516-530, 1965.

7 R. H. Yue, T. Starr, and M. M. Gertler, "The Rivanol Method for the Quantitative Determination of Antithrombin III in Plasma," *Thrombosis et Diathesis Haemorrhagica* 31: 439-451, 1974.

8 W. S. Tillet and R. L. Garner, "The Fibrinolytic Activity of Haemolytic Streptococci," *J. Exp. Med.* 58: 485-502, 1933.

9 L. R. Christensen, "Streptococci Fibrinolysis: A Proteolytic Reaction Due to a Serum Enzyme Activated by Streptococcal Fibrinolysis," *J. Gen. Physiol.* 28: 363-383, 1945.

10 C. R. Rizza, "The Management of Patients With Coagulation Factor Deficiencies," in *Human Blood Coagulation, Haemostasis and Thrombosis,* R. Biggs, ed. (Oxford: Blackwell Scientific Publications, 1972), pp. 333-360.

11 M. M. Gertler, M. A. Woodbury, L. G. Gottsch, P. D. White, and H. A. Rusk, "The Candidate for Coronary Heart Disease," *JAMA* 170: 149-152, 1959.

12 J. R. Hampton and J. R. A. Mitchell, "Abnormalities in Platelet Behaviour in Acute Illnesses," *Brit. Med. J.* 1: 1078-1080, 1966; J. R. Hampton and J. R. A. Mitchell, "Effect of Aggregating Agents on the Electrophoretic Mobility of Human Platelets," *Brit. Med. J.* 1: 1074-1077, 1966; T. H. Spaet and M. B. Zucker, "Mechanism of Platelet Plug Formation and the Role of Adenosine Diphosphate," *Amer. J. Physiol.* 206: 1267-1274, 1964.

13 J. W. Lyttleton, "The Antithrombin Activity of Human Plasma," *Biochem. J.* 58: 8-15, 1954; R. Biggs, K. W. E. Denson, N. Akman et al., "Antithrombin III and Antifactor X_a," *Brit. J. Haemat.* 19: 283-305, 1970.

14 J. R. O'Brien, "Heparin and Platelets," *Cur. Ther. Res.* 18:79-90, 1975.

X Analysis of Risk Factors

Since the physical and biochemical parameters used to classify the individual at risk are based on current research, they are necessarily time-dependent and subject to continual reassessment. This gives the investigation of risk a dynamic quality which, by itself, does not invalidate any one variable or even a set of several variables within a mathematical function. It does, however, stress the need to re-evaluate each new potential risk factor to determine whether it can replace a factor, add to the mathematical function, or both. In this way a more powerful mathematical function—be it a linear model or some other—can be developed to discriminate with greater accuracy the C.H.D.-prone individual.

Coronary heart disease is an evolutionary process that depends largely on time. As a result, the probability of an individual succumbing to the disease is determined by the length of time a single risk factor or concurrent risk factors have been in the abnormal range. Likewise, the ability of the individual to change these risk factors with drugs, new eating habits, and increased physical activity probably changes the variables included in predicting an acute coronary episode. These factors must present themselves in the average time a given profile score remains accurate for the individual. How long this interval is will be a subject for further analysis.

Statistical Analysis

This section describes a specialized method of evaluating certain individual risk factors as they relate to both conditional probability and proportionate risk. In addition,

Table 10.1 Percentage of correctly classified individuals in coronary and control groups for each variable and total profile score

	Coronary group	Control group	Total
Cholesterol	66.1	75.8	72.8
Uric acid	53.8	35.8	41.4
Lipid phosphorus	56.9	57.9	57.6
Height	60.0	62.0	61.4
Mesomorphy	56.9	68.2	64.7
Ectomorphy	66.1	47.5	53.3
Log cholesterol	75.3	48.9	57.1
Log uric acid	75.3	42.7	52.8
Log lipid phosphorus	80.0	31.7	46.6
Log height	86.1	37.2	52.3
Profile score	73.8	74.4	74.2

it offers an over-all assessment of the joint risk factors as a powerful mathematical function that can also be used to assess conditional probability and proportionate risk.

Single-variable analysis

Discriminant functions were developed for single variables. Table 10.1 shows the percentage of coronary subjects and controls who were correctly classified for each variable and for profile score. Each significant variable was determined by an F ratio test. As can be seen in Tables 10.2 through 10.7, when the risk factor probability (determined by the logistic function) increased to greater than the population probability of coronary heart disease (that is, .037 or 3.7 per 100 at age 45), proportionate risk increased and the individual became more susceptible than the average. That was, of course, based on the a priori probability of the population. The logistic function employed was as follows:

$$p = 1/1 + e^{(\log p_1/p_2 \ - \text{ variable score})}$$

where p_2 = probability of C.H.D. = 0.037*

$p_1 = 1 - p_2 \qquad = 0.963$

*Based on statistics in National Center for Health Statistics, Series 11, Number 10, *Coronary Heart Disease in Adults–United States, 1960-1962.* Washington, D.C., 1965.

The following tables and summaries of each variable describe both the risk factor probability, determined by the logistic function, and the proportionate risk. The proportionate risk is the ratio of the risk factor probability to the average risk of 3.7 per 100 of the U.S. male population at age 45. This ratio is the relative risk an individual has of becoming a coronary candidate. For an example of each, consider a lipid phosphorus value of 12.30 mg per cent. The risk factor probability is 0.037, or 3.7 per cent. This represents the same chance of experiencing a coronary episode as the entire male population, or, expressed as a ratio, 1:1. This value is 1.00 in the corresponding proportionate risk column. If the value in this column were to increase to a level above 1.00, the rate of increasing risk of coronary heart disease would be greater than the average male, whereas any proportionate risk below 1.00 confirms a less than average risk rate for the individual.

Serum cholesterol. Serum cholesterol is the major contributor to the over-all risk rate. A serum cholesterol value of 200 mg per cent has a risk factor probability of 1.1×10^{-2} and a proportionate risk of 0.29, or less than three-tenths the risk for the average person. Similarly, a serum cholesterol value of 250 mg per cent has a risk factor probability of 3.4×10^{-2} and a proportionate risk of 0.94. The rates ascend rapidly, giving a serum cholesterol value of 300 a risk factor probability of 1×10^{-1} and a proportionate risk of 2.8 (or 2.8 times more prone to coronary disease). Thus, a rise in serum cholesterol from 200 mg per cent to 300 mg per cent increases one's risk factor probability and one's relative chances of becoming a coronary candidate almost 10-fold (see Table 10.2).

Serum uric acid. Serum uric acid is considered a risk factor, though a less powerful one than serum cholesterol. A serum uric acid of 4.0 mg per cent carries a risk factor probability of 2.4 x 10^{-2} and a proportionate risk of 0.65. A serum uric acid of 4.9 mg per cent increases the risk factor probability to 3.7 x 10^{-2} and the proportionate risk to 1.0 (or an average chance of coronary heart disease). However, a rise in serum uric acid to 8.0 increases the risk probability to 1.5 x 10^{-1} and the proportionate risk to 4.11 (or 4 times greater chance than average). Thus, a twofold increase in serum uric acid will increase the risk factor probability and the probability of becoming a coronary candidate more than 6 times (see Table 10.3). These values are far less than were observed in increases in serum cholesterol values.

Mesomorphy. Mesomorphy carries a risk change with increasing degree. Thus, a value of 3.0 in mesomorphy carries a risk factor probability of 2.0 x 10^{-2} and a proportionate risk of 0.56, or 50 per cent less chance of coming down with heart disease than the average U.S. male. A 5.0 in mesomorphy increases the risk factor probability to 5.6 x 10^{-2} and the proportionate risk to 1.51, increasing proneness to more than 1½ times that of the average male. Mesomorphy of 7.0 carries a risk factor probability of 14.2 x 10^{-2} and a proportionate risk of 3.85. Thus, mesomorphy is almost as powerful a discriminator as serum uric acid (see Table 10.4).

Thus far, only positive parameters have been discussed. But there are negative ones as well—those that mitigate against coronary heart disease. The major negative parameters are discussed below.

Height. Earlier descriptions of the coronary-prone individual described a person of short stature. It is not surprising, therefore, to find that increased height appears to lessen the chances of one's becoming a candidate for coronary heart disease. Thus, a height of 170.48 cm (67 inches) carries a risk factor probability of 3.3 x 10^{-2} and a proportionate risk of 0.91. As height increases to 180.08 cm (71 inches), the risk factor probability decreases to 1.17 x 10^{-2} and the proportionate risk decreases as well to 0.32, or approximately three-tenths of the population average. An extremely tall person of 195.44 cm (77 inches) experiences a further decline in both risk factor probability and proportionate risk to 2.1 x 10^{-3} and 0.06, respectively. Accordingly, an increase of 10 inches produces a factor probability decrease and a relative decrease in the chances of becoming a candidate by 15 times (see Table 10.5).

Ectomorphy. The degree of ectomorphy is to some extent inversely proportionate to the degree of risk, as described in Chapter V. This relationship is apparent in Table 10.6. Thus, as ectomorphy increases from 3.0, to 5.0, to 7.0, the risk factor probability decreases from 3.2 x 10^{-2}, to 1.8 x 10^{-2}, to 1.0 x 10^{-2}, respectively. Similarly, the chances of an individual becoming a candidate for coronary heart disease decreases from 89.1 x 10^{-2}, to 50.7 x 10^{-2}, to 28.6 x 10^{-2}, respectively, indicating a decreasing risk of from less than nine-tenths of the population average to less than three-tenths of the population average.

Each of these risk factors should be considered independently of the others. Their contiguous nature, though strongly indicative of the possibility of future cardiovascular disease, does not consider the multiple interrelationships existing between these significant risk factors. Thus, a more powerful or accurate predictor of coronary candidacy is the multiple-variable discriminant function.

The pre-eminence of this approach is shown with serum lipid phosphorus.

Lipid phosphorus. This variable, considered alone, increases risk as it rises in value. A serum lipid phosphorus value of 8.0 mg per cent (phospholipids of 200 mg per cent) produces a risk factor probability of 2.0×10^{-2} and a proportionate risk of 0.54, which is a little more than half the risk to the average male. An increase in serum lipid phosphorus to 14.0 mg per cent (phospholipids of 350 mg per cent) raises the risk factor probability to 4.7×10^{-2} and proportionate risk to 1.27:1 (see Table 10.7).

The literature establishes that phospholipids are antagonistic to cholesterol in many biological reactions. However, the contribution of lipid phosphorus as a protective agent is only demonstrated within the framework of multiple-variable analysis. This is shown by the negative risk rate of the variable in the multiple function to follow. Thus, the diametric opposition encountered with regard to the risk rate of lipid phosphorus is seen not as a contradiction but as a natural progression of the variable from a single risk factor to a member of a multiple interrelationship.

Multiple-variable analysis

A discriminant function analysis was performed on those variables considered to contribute the most to increased risk of coronary heart disease. The variables were chosen from the previous linear regression analysis (see Chapter II). Seventy-four and two-tenths per cent of the individuals were correctly classified from this analysis. The order in which the variables were entered into the regression is shown below, along with coefficients. The formula for the profile score also appears.

	C_i
Log cholesterol	9.59
Family history of siblings	3.49
Mesomorphy	0.432
Log height	–8.86
Family history of father	0.233
Log uric acid	3.91
Log lipid phosphorus	–2.73
Family history of mother	0.125
Constant C_0	–5.96

Profile score value = 9.59 (log cholesterol) + 3.49 (positive FH siblings) + 0.432 (mesomorphy) – 8.86 (log height) + 0.233 (positive FH father) + 3.91 (log uric acid) – 2.73 (log lipid phosphorus) + 0.125 (positive FH mother) – 5.96 (constant).

Another discriminant function was calculated using the six most discriminating variables from the above analysis, that is, log cholesterol, log uric acid, log height, log lipid phosphorus, history of heart disease in siblings, and mesomorphy. With these six variables the grand means were inserted, thus allowing more subjects to be included in the formulation of a profile score. An F ratio test was used to determine which of the six variables were to be included. The four variables chosen as significant are listed below with their coefficients and the formula for the profile score.

	C_i	$\times$ σ_x	= Standardized coefficient
Log cholesterol (mg. %)	11.05	0.092	= 1.014
Positive family history of siblings*	1.78	0.423	= 0.757
Log uric acid (mg. %)	5.13	0.084	= 0.431
Log height (inches)	–33.70	0.016	= 0.528
Constant term	31.38		

Profile score = 11.05 (log cholesterol) – 33.70 (log height) + 5.13 (log uric acid) + 1.78 (positive FH siblings) + 31.38 (constant)

*Positive FH of siblings 0 = no presence of C.H.D.
1 = presence of C.H.D.

The value obtained by multiplying the coefficient by its standard deviation permits one to assess the contribution made by each variable. Cholesterol discriminates the best followed by positive history of C.H.D. in siblings, height, and uric acid. This discriminant function correctly classified 79.8 per cent of our subjects.

Considering the prevalence of definite and suspected coronary heart disease in U.S. males (3.7 per 100), the conditional probabilities and proportionate risks shown in Table 10.8 were obtained using the following multiple logistic function:

$$p = 1/1 + e^{(\log p_1/p_2 \; - \; \text{profile score})}$$

where p_2 = probability of C.H.D. = 0.037

$p_1 = 1 - p_2$ = 0.963

The data in Table 10.8 indicate the chances of an individual developing coronary heart disease in terms of proportionate risk. Thus, a person with a profile score of –9.0 has a 52.4 x 10^{-7} conditional probability of having an acute myocardial infarction, compared with the average risk of 3.7 x 10^{-2} at age 45. Interpreted another way, the profile score of –9.0 would indicate a proportionate risk of 1 in 10,000 for an acute coronary event. Similarly, a profile score of 5.0 would indicate a conditional probability of 86.3 x 10^{-2}, or 23.3 times the chance of having an acute coronary event as the average person of similar age. Figure 10.1 shows the sigmoid curve of the conditional probability based on profile score.

To further elucidate the strong predictive power of serum cholesterol on mortality rates, the original cholesterol values of the coronary group were compared. The results of the analysis did not demonstrate an all-or-none survival with respect to "threshold" levels of serum cholesterol.

Table 10.9 compares coronary subjects whose serum cholesterol was below 220 mg per cent with subjects whose cholesterol levels were above 220 mg per cent, for the first 10 years of survival. In the fourth year there was a significant difference between the 260-299 mg per cent and 300-339 mg per cent groups and the <220 mg per cent group.

Table 10.2 Risk factor probability and proportionate risk for increasing degrees of cholesterol (mg. %)

Variable value	Risk factor probability	Proportionate risk
140.00	0.002756	0.074474
141.00	0.002820	0.076229
142.00	0.002887	0.078026
143.00	0.002955	0.079864
144.00	0.003025	0.081746
145.00	0.003096	0.083672
146.00	0.003169	0.085643
147.00	0.003243	0.087661
148.00	0.003320	0.089726
149.00	0.003398	0.091840
150.00	0.003478	0.094003
151.00	0.003560	0.096216
152.00	0.003644	0.098482
153.00	0.003730	0.100801
154.00	0.003817	0.103175
155.00	0.003907	0.105603
156.00	0.003999	0.108089
157.00	0.004093	0.110634
158.00	0.004190	0.113238
159.00	0.004288	0.115902
160.00	0.004389	0.118630
161.00	0.004493	0.121421
162.00	0.004598	0.124277
163.00	0.004706	0.127201
164.00	0.004817	0.130193
165.00	0.004930	0.133255
166.00	0.005046	0.136388
167.00	0.005165	0.139595
168.00	0.005286	0.142877
169.00	0.005411	0.146236
170.00	0.005538	0.149673
171.00	0.005668	0.153190
172.00	0.005801	0.156790
173.00	0.005938	0.160474
174.00	0.006077	0.164244
175.00	0.006220	0.168101
176.00	0.006366	0.172049
177.00	0.006515	0.176089
178.00	0.006668	0.180223
179.00	0.006825	0.184454
180.00	0.006985	0.188783
181.00	0.007149	0.193213
182.00	0.007317	0.197746
183.00	0.007488	0.202385
184.00	0.007664	0.207131
185.00	0.007844	0.211988
186.00	0.008027	0.216959
187.00	0.008216	0.222044
188.00	0.008408	0.227248
189.00	0.008605	0.232573
190.00	0.008807	0.238021
191.00	0.009013	0.243596
192.00	0.009224	0.249301

Variable value	Risk factor probability	Proportionate risk
193.00	0.009440	0.255137
194.00	0.009661	0.261109
195.00	0.009887	0.267220
196.00	0.010118	0.273471
197.00	0.010355	0.279868
198.00	0.010597	0.286412
199.00	0.010845	0.293108
200.00	0.011098	0.299959
201.00	0.011358	0.306968
202.00	0.011623	0.314139
203.00	0.011895	0.321475
204.00	0.012172	0.328981
205.00	0.012456	0.336659
206.00	0.012747	0.344515
207.00	0.013044	0.352552
208.00	0.013349	0.360773
209.00	0.013660	0.369183
210.00	0.013978	0.377787
211.00	0.014304	0.386588
212.00	0.014637	0.395591
213.00	0.014978	0.404801
214.00	0.015326	0.414222
215.00	0.015683	0.423858
216.00	0.016047	0.433716
217.00	0.016421	0.443798
218.00	0.016802	0.454111
219.00	0.017192	0.464659
220.00	0.017592	0.475449
221.00	0.018000	0.486483
222.00	0.018417	0.497770
223.00	0.018845	0.509313
224.00	0.019281	0.521118
225.00	0.019728	0.533192
226.00	0.020185	0.545539
227.00	0.020652	0.558167
228.00	0.021130	0.571081
229.00	0.021619	0.584286
230.00	0.022118	0.597790
231.00	0.022629	0.611599
232.00	0.023152	0.625720
233.00	0.023686	0.640159
234.00	0.024232	0.654922
235.00	0.024791	0.670017
236.00	0.025362	0.685452
237.00	0.025946	0.701232
238.00	0.026543	0.717365
239.00	0.027153	0.733860
240.00	0.027777	0.750723
241.00	0.028415	0.767962
242.00	0.029067	0.785586
243.00	0.029733	0.803601
244.00	0.030415	0.822016
245.00	0.031111	0.840840

Variable value	Risk factor probability	Proportionate risk	Variable value	Risk factor probability	Proportionate risk
246.00	0.031823	0.860081	293.00	0.089700	2.424318
247.00	0.032551	0.879747	294.00	0.091626	2.476365
248.00	0.033294	0.899848	295.00	0.093588	2.529418
249.00	0.034054	0.920391	296.00	0.095589	2.583486
250.00	0.034831	0.941387	297.00	0.097628	2.638586
251.00	0.035625	0.962844	298.00	0.099705	2.694731
252.00	0.036437	0.984772	299.00	0.101822	2.751935
253.00	0.037266	1.007178	300.00	0.103978	2.810215
254.00	0.038113	1.030077	301.00	0.106175	2.869583
255.00	0.038979	1.053473	302.00	0.108412	2.930052
256.00	0.039863	1.077380	303.00	0.110691	2.991637
257.00	0.040767	1.101806	304.00	0.113011	3.054355
258.00	0.041690	1.126761	305.00	0.115374	3.118214
259.00	0.042634	1.152257	306.00	0.117780	3.183234
260.00	0.043597	1.178302	307.00	0.120229	3.249424
261.00	0.044582	1.204909	308.00	0.122722	3.316800
262.00	0.045587	1.232090	309.00	0.125259	3.385371
263.00	0.046615	1.259853	310.00	0.127841	3.455157
264.00	0.047664	1.288210	311.00	0.130468	3.526166
265.00	0.048735	1.317174	312.00	0.133141	3.598412
266.00	0.049830	1.346754	313.00	0.135860	3.671902
267.00	0.050948	1.376963	314.00	0.138626	3.746657
268.00	0.052089	1.407811	315.00	0.141439	3.822686
269.00	0.053255	1.439313	316.00	0.144300	3.899998
270.00	0.054445	1.471480	317.00	0.147208	3.978603
271.00	0.055660	1.504323	318.00	0.150165	4.058518
272.00	0.056901	1.537853	319.00	0.153171	4.139750
273.00	0.058167	1.572086	320.00	0.156225	4.222307
274.00	0.059460	1.607035	321.00	0.159329	4.306199
275.00	0.060780	1.642708	322.00	0.162483	4.391439
276.00	0.062127	1.679121	323.00	0.165687	4.478036
277.00	0.063503	1.716285	324.00	0.168942	4.565991
278.00	0.064906	1.754217	325.00	0.172247	4.655321
279.00	0.066338	1.792927	326.00	0.175603	4.746030
280.00	0.067800	1.832430	327.00	0.179011	4.83812[illegible]
281.00	0.069291	1.872739	328.00	0.182469	4.931602
282.00	0.070813	1.913868	329.00	0.185980	5.026484
283.00	0.072366	1.955826	330.00	0.189542	5.122769
284.00	0.073950	1.998635	331.00	0.193157	5.220460
285.00	0.075565	2.042303	332.00	0.196824	5.319556
286.00	0.077213	2.086847	333.00	0.200543	5.420073
287.00	0.078894	2.132277	334.00	0.204314	5.522003
288.00	0.080609	2.178611	335.00	0.208138	5.625353
289.00	0.082357	2.225863	336.00	0.212014	5.730117
290.00	0.084140	2.274042	337.00	0.215943	5.836303
291.00	0.085957	2.323170	338.00	0.219925	5.943909
292.00	0.087811	2.373257	339.00	0.223958	6.052927

Table 10.3 Risk factor probability and proportionate risk for increasing degrees of uric acid (mg. %)

Variable value	Risk factor probability	Proportionate risk	Variable value	Risk factor probability	Proportionate risk
3.00	0.014845	0.401228	6.00	0.062522	1.689780
3.10	0.015588	0.421305	6.10	0.065492	1.770048
3.20	0.016368	0.442370	6.20	0.068592	1.853848
3.30	0.017185	0.464469	6.30	0.071829	1.941314
3.40	0.018043	0.487652	6.40	0.075205	2.032570
3.50	0.018943	0.511971	6.50	0.078727	2.127751
3.60	0.019887	0.537477	6.60	0.082399	2.226996
3.70	0.020876	0.564226	6.70	0.086226	2.330435
3.80	0.021914	0.592278	6.80	0.090214	2.438207
3.90	0.023003	0.621692	6.90	0.094367	2.550447
4.00	0.024144	0.652530	7.00	0.098690	2.667295
4.10	0.025340	0.684858	7.10	0.103189	2.788883
4.20	0.026594	0.718744	7.20	0.107868	2.915352
4.30	0.027908	0.754258	7.30	0.112733	3.046836
4.40	0.029285	0.791475	7.40	0.117788	3.183466
4.50	0.030727	0.830470	7.50	0.123039	3.325377
4.60	0.032239	0.871323	7.60	0.128489	3.472688
4.70	0.033822	0.914115	7.70	0.134145	3.625529
4.80	0.035480	0.958931	7.80	0.140009	3.784014
4.90	0.037217	1.005859	7.90	0.146086	3.948258
5.00	0.039035	1.054993	8.00	0.152380	4.118372
5.10	0.040938	1.106423	8.10	0.158895	4.294447
5.20	0.042929	1.160250	8.20	0.165634	4.476583
5.30	0.045013	1.216571	8.30	0.172600	4.664854
5.40	0.047193	1.275491	8.40	0.179796	4.859341
5.50	0.049473	1.337118	8.50	0.187224	5.060098
5.60	0.051858	1.401560	8.60	0.194886	5.267179
5.70	0.054350	1.468929	8.70	0.202783	5.480623
5.80	0.056956	1.539344	8.80	0.210917	5.700448
5.90	0.059678	1.612922	8.90	0.219287	5.926667

Table 10.4 Risk factor probability and proportionate risk for increasing degrees of mesomorphy

Variable value	Risk factor probability	Proportionate risk	Variable value	Risk factor probability	Proportionate risk
0.10	0.004805	0.129871	1.40	0.009316	0.251779
0.20	0.005057	0.136669	1.50	0.009801	0.264895
0.30	0.005321	0.143821	1.60	0.010311	0.278687
0.40	0.005600	0.151345	1.70	0.010848	0.293190
0.50	0.005893	0.159261	1.80	0.011412	0.308439
0.60	0.006201	0.167588	1.90	0.012005	0.324471
0.70	0.006525	0.176347	2.00	0.012629	0.341326
0.80	0.006866	0.185561	2.10	0.013285	0.359044
0.90	0.007224	0.195253	2.20	0.013974	0.377670
1.00	0.007602	0.205447	2.30	0.014698	0.397247
1.10	0.007998	0.216169	2.40	0.015459	0.417823
1.20	0.008415	0.227446	2.50	0.016260	0.439447
1.30	0.008854	0.239306	2.60	0.017100	0.462172

Variable value	Risk factor probability	Proportionate risk	Variable value	Risk factor probability	Proportionate risk
2.70	0.017984	0.486049	4.90	0.053549	1.447259
2.80	0.018912	0.511137	5.00	0.056208	1.519122
2.90	0.019887	0.537493	5.10	0.058990	1.594328
3.00	0.020912	0.565179	5.20	0.061902	1.673014
3.10	0.021988	0.594260	5.30	0.064947	1.755315
3.20	0.023118	0.624801	5.40	0.068131	1.841370
3.30	0.024304	0.656873	5.50	0.071459	1.931322
3.40	0.025550	0.690549	5.60	0.074937	2.025314
3.50	0.026858	0.725903	5.70	0.078569	2.123496
3.60	0.028232	0.763014	5.80	0.082362	2.226012
3.70	0.029673	0.801966	5.90	0.086321	2.333013
3.80	0.031185	0.842841	6.00	0.090452	2.444652
3.90	0.032772	0.885730	6.10	0.094760	2.561078
4.00	0.034437	0.930724	6.20	0.099250	2.682444
4.10	0.036183	0.977917	6.30	0.103929	2.808899
4.20	0.038014	1.027410	6.40	0.108802	2.940598
4.30	0.039934	1.079304	6.50	0.113874	3.077689
4.40	0.041947	1.133704	6.60	0.119152	3.220311
4.50	0.044057	1.190721	6.70	0.124639	3.368617
4.60	0.046267	1.250467	6.80	0.130341	3.522739
4.70	0.048583	1.313058	6.90	0.136264	3.682819
4.80	0.051009	1.378613	7.00	0.142412	3.848981

Table 10.5 Risk factor probability and proportionate risk for increasing height (cm .)

Variable value	Risk factor probability	Proportionate risk	Variable value	Risk factor probability	Proportionate risk
150.00	0.255603	6.908185	165.36	0.058066	1.569347
150.64	0.242226	6.546651	166.00	0.054274	1.466867
151.28	0.229334	6.198208	166.64	0.050716	1.370699
151.92	0.216934	5.863072	167.28	0.047379	1.280519
152.56	0.205023	5.541168	167.92	0.044253	1.196013
153.20	0.193607	5.232634	168.56	0.041323	1.116827
153.84	0.182679	4.937270	169.20	0.038579	1.042671
154.48	0.172236	4.655015	169.84	0.036011	0.973269
155.12	0.162273	4.385750	170.48	0.033607	0.908311
155.76	0.152778	4.129132	171.12	0.031359	0.847547
156.40	0.143743	3.884953	171.76	0.029257	0.790737
157.04	0.135159	3.652959	172.40	0.027292	0.737617
157.68	0.127011	3.432716	173.04	0.025455	0.687972
158.32	0.119285	3.223922	173.68	0.023739	0.641595
158.96	0.111971	3.026238	174.32	0.022136	0.598266
159.60	0.105050	2.839194	174.96	0.020639	0.557801
160.24	0.098510	2.662427	175.60	0.019241	0.520026
160.88	0.092336	2.495564	176.24	0.017936	0.484756
161.52	0.086511	2.338122	176.88	0.016718	0.451844
162.16	0.081021	2.189758	177.52	0.015582	0.421124
162.80	0.075850	2.049998	178.16	0.014521	0.392462
163.44	0.070983	1.918468	178.80	0.013532	0.365730
164.08	0.066408	1.794797	179.44	0.012609	0.340790
164.72	0.062106	1.678542	180.08	0.011749	0.317531

Variable value	Risk factor probability	Proportionate risk	Variable value	Risk factor probability	Proportionate risk
180.72	0.010946	0.295845	190.96	0.003510	0.094858
181.36	0.010198	0.275622	191.60	0.003268	0.088330
182.00	0.009500	0.256767	192.24	0.003043	0.082248
182.64	0.008850	0.239195	192.88	0.002834	0.076584
183.28	0.008244	0.222811	193.52	0.002638	0.071310
183.92	0.007679	0.207542	194.16	0.002457	0.066397
184.56	0.007153	0.193314	194.80	0.002287	0.061822
185.20	0.006662	0.180052	195.44	0.002130	0.057562
185.84	0.006205	0.167694	196.08	0.001983	0.053595
186.48	0.005779	0.156182	196.72	0.001846	0.049900
187.12	0.005382	0.145453	197.36	0.001719	0.046461
187.76	0.005012	0.135458	198.00	0.001601	0.043257
188.40	0.004668	0.126149	198.64	0.001490	0.040274
189.04	0.004347	0.117474	199.28	0.001387	0.037497
189.68	0.004048	0.109396	199.92	0.001292	0.034911
190.32	0.003769	0.101869	200.56	0.001203	0.032503

Table 10.6 Risk factor probability and proportionate risk for increasing degrees of ectomorphy

Variable value	Risk factor probability	Proportionate risk	Variable value	Risk factor probability	Proportionate risk
0.10	0.073239	1.979433	3.10	0.032082	0.867077
0.20	0.071297	1.926953	3.20	0.031195	0.843097
0.30	0.069403	1.875761	3.30	0.030331	0.819758
0.40	0.067556	1.825830	3.40	0.029491	0.797046
0.50	0.065754	1.777135	3.50	0.028673	0.774945
0.60	0.063997	1.729648	3.60	0.027877	0.753439
0.70	0.062284	1.683347	3.70	0.027103	0.732513
0.80	0.060614	1.638205	3.80	0.026350	0.712153
0.90	0.058985	1.594196	3.90	0.025617	0.692343
1.00	0.057398	1.551298	4.00	0.024904	0.673071
1.10	0.055851	1.509486	4.10	0.024210	0.654321
1.20	0.054343	1.468735	4.20	0.023535	0.636081
1.30	0.052874	1.429023	4.30	0.022879	0.618338
1.40	0.051442	1.390326	4.40	0.022240	0.601079
1.50	0.050047	1.352622	4.50	0.021619	0.584291
1.60	0.048688	1.315888	4.60	0.021015	0.567961
1.70	0.047364	1.280102	4.70	0.020427	0.552078
1.80	0.046074	1.245243	4.80	0.019855	0.536631
1.90	0.044818	1.211287	4.90	0.019299	0.521607
2.00	0.043594	1.178215	5.00	0.018759	0.506995
2.10	0.042402	1.146006	5.10	0.018233	0.492786
2.20	0.041242	1.114639	5.20	0.017722	0.478967
2.30	0.040112	1.084095	5.30	0.017225	0.465529
2.40	0.039011	1.054355	5.40	0.016741	0.452463
2.50	0.037940	1.025397	5.50	0.016271	0.439756
2.60	0.036897	0.997205	5.60	0.015814	0.427401
2.70	0.035881	0.969759	5.70	0.015369	0.415387
2.80	0.034893	0.943041	5.80	0.014937	0.403705
2.90	0.033930	0.917033	5.90	0.014517	0.392348
3.00	0.032994	0.891717	6.00	0.014108	0.381305

Variable value	Risk factor probability	Proportionate risk	Variable value	Risk factor probability	Proportionate risk
6.10	0.013711	0.370569	6.60	0.011885	0.321204
6.20	0.013325	0.360131	6.70	0.011549	0.312140
6.30	0.012949	0.349984	6.80	0.011223	0.303329
6.40	0.012584	0.340118	6.90	0.010906	0.294764
6.50	0.012230	0.330527	7.00	0.010598	0.286439

Table 10.7 Risk factor probability and proportionate risk for increasing degrees of lipid phosphorus (mg. %)

Variable value	Risk factor probability	Proportionate risk	Variable value	Risk factor probability	Proportionate risk
6.00	0.015051	0.406784	10.10	0.027114	0.732817
6.10	0.015270	0.412698	10.20	0.027504	0.743339
6.20	0.015492	0.418698	10.30	0.027898	0.754008
6.30	0.015717	0.424782	10.40	0.028299	0.764826
6.40	0.015945	0.430954	10.50	0.028704	0.775794
6.50	0.016177	0.437214	10.60	0.029116	0.786915
6.60	0.016412	0.443564	10.70	0.029533	0.798191
6.70	0.016650	0.450004	10.80	0.029956	0.809623
6.80	0.016892	0.456536	10.90	0.030385	0.821213
6.90	0.017137	0.463161	11.00	0.030820	0.832965
7.00	0.017386	0.469881	11.10	0.031261	0.844879
7.10	0.017638	0.476696	11.20	0.031707	0.856958
7.20	0.017894	0.483608	11.30	0.032161	0.869204
7.30	0.018153	0.490619	11.40	0.032620	0.881620
7.40	0.018416	0.497729	11.50	0.033086	0.894206
7.50	0.018683	0.504941	11.60	0.033558	0.906966
7.60	0.018953	0.512256	11.70	0.034036	0.919901
7.70	0.019228	0.519673	11.80	0.034522	0.933015
7.80	0.019506	0.527196	11.90	0.035013	0.946308
7.90	0.019789	0.534826	12.00	0.035512	0.959784
8.00	0.020075	0.542565	12.10	0.036017	0.973445
8.10	0.020365	0.550412	12.20	0.036530	0.987293
8.20	0.020660	0.558371	12.30	0.037049	1.001329
8.30	0.020958	0.566443	12.40	0.037576	1.015558
8.40	0.021261	0.574629	12.50	0.038109	1.029982
8.50	0.021568	0.582930	12.60	0.038650	1.044601
8.60	0.021880	0.591348	12.70	0.039199	1.059421
8.70	0.022196	0.599886	12.80	0.039754	1.074442
8.80	0.022516	0.608544	12.90	0.040318	1.089665
8.90	0.022841	0.617324	13.00	0.040889	1.105097
9.00	0.023170	0.626227	13.10	0.041467	1.120737
9.10	0.023504	0.635256	13.20	0.042054	1.136589
9.20	0.023843	0.644412	13.30	0.042648	1.152655
9.30	0.024187	0.653697	13.40	0.043251	1.168938
9.40	0.024535	0.663112	13.50	0.043861	1.185440
9.50	0.024888	0.672659	13.60	0.044480	1.202165
9.60	0.025247	0.682340	13.70	0.045107	1.219113
9.70	0.025610	0.692157	13.80	0.045743	1.236289
9.80	0.025978	0.702111	13.90	0.046387	1.253697
9.90	0.026352	0.712204	14.00	0.047040	1.271338
10.00	0.026730	0.722439	14.10	0.047701	1.289211

Variable value	Risk factor probability	Proportionate risk	Variable value	Risk factor probability	Proportionate risk
14.20	0.048371	1.307326	15.10	0.054818	1.481565
14.30	0.049050	1.325683	15.20	0.055582	1.502226
14.40	0.049738	1.344282	15.30	0.056357	1.523156
14.50	0.050436	1.363130	15.40	0.057141	1.544359
14.60	0.051142	1.382226	15.50	0.057936	1.565842
14.70	0.051858	1.401577	15.60	0.058741	1.587604
14.80	0.052584	1.421183	15.70	0.059557	1.609649
14.90	0.053319	1.441049	15.80	0.060383	1.631980
15.00	0.054063	1.461174	15.90	0.061220	1.654600

Table 10.8 Conditional probability and proportionate risk with increasing profile score (−9.0 to +8.9)

Profile score	Conditional probability	Proportionate risk	Profile score	Conditional probability	Proportionate risk
−9.0	0.00000524	0.0001	−5.3	0.00021191	0.0057
−8.9	0.00000579	0.0002	−5.2	0.00023420	0.0063
−8.8	0.00000640	0.0002	−5.1	0.00025882	0.0070
−8.7	0.00000707	0.0002	−5.0	0.00028603	0.0077
−8.6	0.00000782	0.0002	−4.9	0.00031611	0.0085
−8.5	0.00000864	0.0002	−4.8	0.00034934	0.0094
−8.4	0.00000955	0.0003	−4.7	0.00038606	0.0104
−8.3	0.00001055	0.0003	−4.6	0.00042665	0.0115
−8.2	0.00001166	0.0003	−4.5	0.00047150	0.0127
−8.1	0.00001289	0.0003	−4.4	0.00052106	0.0141
−8.0	0.00001424	0.0004	−4.3	0.00057583	0.0156
−7.9	0.00001574	0.0004	−4.2	0.00063636	0.0172
−7.8	0.00001740	0.0005	−4.1	0.00070323	0.0190
−7.7	0.00001923	0.0005	−4.0	0.00077714	0.0210
−7.6	0.00002125	0.0006	−3.9	0.00085880	0.0232
−7.5	0.00002348	0.0006	−3.8	0.00094904	0.0256
−7.4	0.00002595	0.0007	−3.7	0.00104874	0.0283
−7.3	0.00002868	0.0008	−3.6	0.00115891	0.0313
−7.2	0.00003170	0.0009	−3.5	0.00128064	0.0346
−7.1	0.00003504	0.0009	−3.4	0.00141514	0.0382
−7.0	0.00003872	0.0010	−3.3	0.00156373	0.0423
−6.9	0.00004279	0.0012	−3.2	0.00172791	0.0467
−6.8	0.00004729	0.0013	−3.1	0.00190929	0.0516
−6.7	0.00005227	0.0014	−3.0	0.00210967	0.0570
−6.6	0.00005776	0.0016	−2.9	0.00233103	0.0630
−6.5	0.00006384	0.0017	−2.8	0.00257555	0.0696
−6.4	0.00007055	0.0019	−2.7	0.00284566	0.0769
−6.3	0.00007797	0.0021	−2.6	0.00314400	0.0850
−6.2	0.00008617	0.0023	−2.5	0.00347351	0.0939
−6.1	0.00009523	0.0026	−2.4	0.00383742	0.1037
−6.0	0.00010524	0.0028	−2.3	0.00423929	0.1146
−5.9	0.00011631	0.0031	−2.2	0.00468306	0.1266
−5.8	0.00012854	0.0035	−2.1	0.00517303	0.1398
−5.7	0.00014206	0.0038	−2.0	0.00571398	0.1544
−5.6	0.00015700	0.0042	−1.9	0.00631114	0.1706
−5.5	0.00017351	0.0047	−1.8	0.00697026	0.1884
−5.4	0.00019175	0.0052	−1.7	0.00769769	0.2080

Profile score	Conditional probability	Proportionate risk	Profile score	Conditional probability	Proportion risk
−1.6	0.00850039	0.2297	3.7	0.63201684	17.0815
−1.5	0.00938599	0.2537	3.8	0.65495187	17.7014
−1.4	0.01036290	0.2801	3.9	0.67718744	18.3024
−1.3	0.01144031	0.3092	4.0	0.69864959	18.8824
−1.2	0.01262831	0.3413	4.1	0.71927673	19.4399
−1.1	0.01393794	0.3767	4.2	0.73901874	19.9735
−1.0	0.01538126	0.4157	4.3	0.75784034	20.4822
−0.9	0.01697146	0.4587	4.4	0.77571625	20.9653
−0.8	0.01872296	0.5060	4.5	0.79263371	21.4225
−0.7	0.02065139	0.5581	4.6	0.80858976	21.8538
−0.6	0.02277386	0.6155	4.7	0.82359141	22.2592
−0.5	0.02510886	0.6786	4.8	0.83765388	22.6393
−0.4	0.02767649	0.7480	4.9	0.85079783	22.9945
−0.3	0.03049850	0.8243	5.0	0.86305177	23.3257
−0.2	0.03359826	0.9081	5.1	0.87444800	23.6337
−0.1	0.03700109	1.0000	5.2	0.88502210	23.9195
0.0	0.04073400	1.1009	5.3	0.89481229	24.1841
0.1	0.04482602	1.2115	5.4	0.90385985	24.4286
0.2	0.04930792	1.3326	5.5	0.91220576	24.6542
0.3	0.05421257	1.4652	5.6	0.91989142	24.8619
0.4	0.05957450	1.6101	5.7	0.92695814	25.0529
0.5	0.06542999	1.7684	5.8	0.93344569	25.2283
0.6	0.07181716	1.9410	5.9	0.93939567	25.3891
0.7	0.07877517	2.1291	6.0	0.94484520	25.5363
0.8	0.08634472	2.3336	6.1	0.94983065	25.6711
0.9	0.09456682	2.5559	6.2	0.95438659	25.7942
1.0	0.10348320	2.7968	6.3	0.95854729	25.9067
1.1	0.11313528	3.0577	6.4	0.96234417	26.0093
1.2	0.12356353	3.3396	6.5	0.96580458	26.1028
1.3	0.13480693	3.6434	6.6	0.96895766	26.1880
1.4	0.14690191	3.9703	6.7	0.97182870	26.2656
1.5	0.15988147	4.3211	6.8	0.97444141	26.3362
1.6	0.17377424	4.6966	6.9	0.97681701	26.4005
1.7	0.18860328	5.0974	7.0	0.97897661	26.4588
1.8	0.20438462	5.5239	7.1	0.98093921	26.5119
1.9	0.22112668	5.9764	7.2	0.98272181	26.5600
2.0	0.23882848	6.4548	7.3	0.98433989	26.6038
2.1	0.25747889	6.9589	7.4	0.98580950	26.6435
2.2	0.27705556	7.4880	7.5	0.98714215	26.6795
2.3	0.29752427	8.0412	7.6	0.98835176	26.7122
2.4	0.31883836	8.6173	7.7	0.98944849	26.7419
2.5	0.34093821	9.2145	7.8	0.99044293	26.7687
2.6	0.36375189	9.8311	7.9	0.99134463	26.7931
2.7	0.38719529	10.4647	8.0	0.99216163	26.8152
2.8	0.41117316	11.1128	8.1	0.99290293	26.8352
2.9	0.43558049	11.7724	8.2	0.99357373	26.8533
3.0	0.46030408	12.4407	8.3	0.99418133	26.8698
3.1	0.48522449	13.1142	8.4	0.99473304	26.8847
3.2	0.51021868	13.7897	8.5	0.99523157	26.8981
3.3	0.53516191	14.4638	8.6	0.99568325	26.9104
3.4	0.55993032	15.1333	8.7	0.99609286	26.9214
3.5	0.58440417	15.7947	8.8	0.99646294	26.9314
3.6	0.60846835	16.4451	8.9	0.99679828	26.9405

In the fifth, sixth, and seventh year survival periods there were significant differences between the >340 mg per cent and the <220 mg per cent groups. The trends revealed in Table 10.9 are graphically illustrated in Figure 10.2, which represents the five-point moving average of survival rates for the various cholesterol categories.

Table 10.10 compares the long-term survival rates of coronary subjects with varying levels of cholesterol ("long-term" meaning 20 years or longer). It can be seen that after 20 years' survival there were significant differences between the coronary subjects with serum cholesterol <220 mg per cent and those with serum cholesterol at various levels above 220 mg per cent. Table 10.11 summarizes these findings and compares the survival rates for cholesterol levels above and below 300 mg per cent. Again, a significant difference between these two groups can be seen in terms of long-term survival. Figure 10.3 graphically shows the survival rates of these two groups.

Other Risk Factors

There are other risk factors associated with heart disease which, while they do not appear to be as influential as the aforementioned, should nevertheless be noted. They include diabetes mellitus, psychological influences, and cigarette smoking.

Diabetes mellitus

There is ample evidence to suggest that atherosclerosis advances more rapidly in individuals with diabetes mellitus than in nondiabetics.[1] In fact, there is some indication that an overtreated diabetic—one who has received more insulin than is required—develops atherosclerosis faster than a diabetic who goes undertreated (as judged by the presence of moderate glucosuria but no acetonemia).[2]

One can only conclude that a disturbance of glucose metabolism, including insulin, is associated with an increase in atherosclerosis to a statistically significant degree. In several studies diabetes mellitus has been considered to be an independent variable.

The relationship between serum triglycerides, immunoreactive insulin, and carbohydrate metabolism in both coronary heart disease subjects and controls has been a subject of discussion.[3] This relationship is particularly strong in individuals with type IV lipoproteinemia in which triglycerides are elevated and where diabetes mellitus exists in about 40 per cent of the cases. Gertler and colleagues studied this subject,[4] accumulating data on two groups: (a) men with coronary heart disease and their age-matched controls and (b) men with ischemic thrombotic cerebrovascular disease and age-matched controls. Table 10.12 is a summary of the published data and Table 10.13 summarizes the percentage of abnormal and normal glucose tolerance responses following an oral glucose tolerance test (G.T.T.) in which 75 grams were administered in the form of Glucola.

It is apparent from this table that the number of abnormal G.T.T.s was significantly higher in the men with ischemic thrombotic cerebrovascular disease but not in the men with coronary heart disease.

The observations about serum immunoreactive insulin (IRI) responses are revealing as well (see Table 10.14). These data show that the response in the ITCVD group was sui generis. The IRI rose rapidly during the first hour, reached its peak at two hours, and

Figure 10.1 Sigmoid curve of the conditional probability based upon profile score

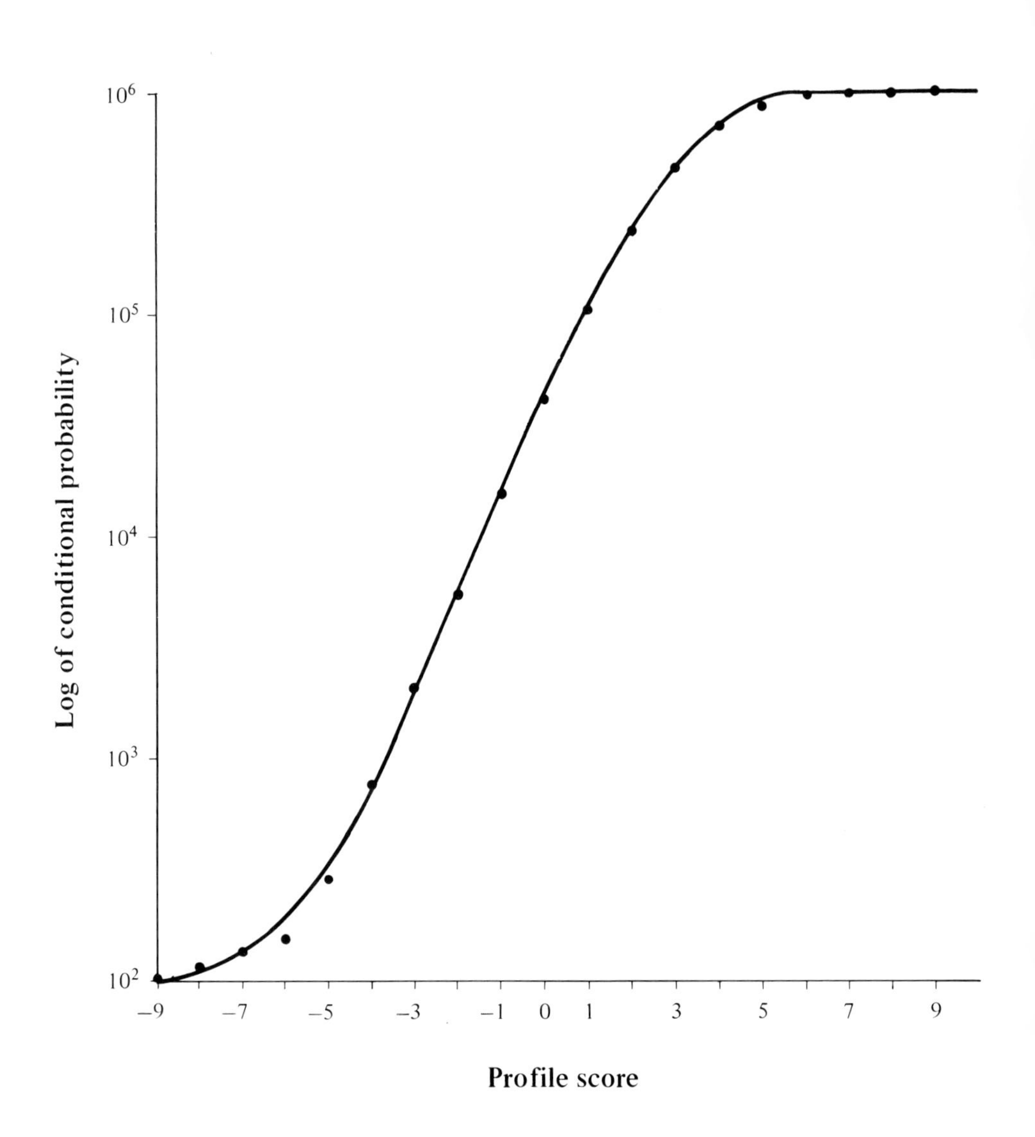

Figure 10.2 Five-point moving average of survival rates for various degrees of cholesterol

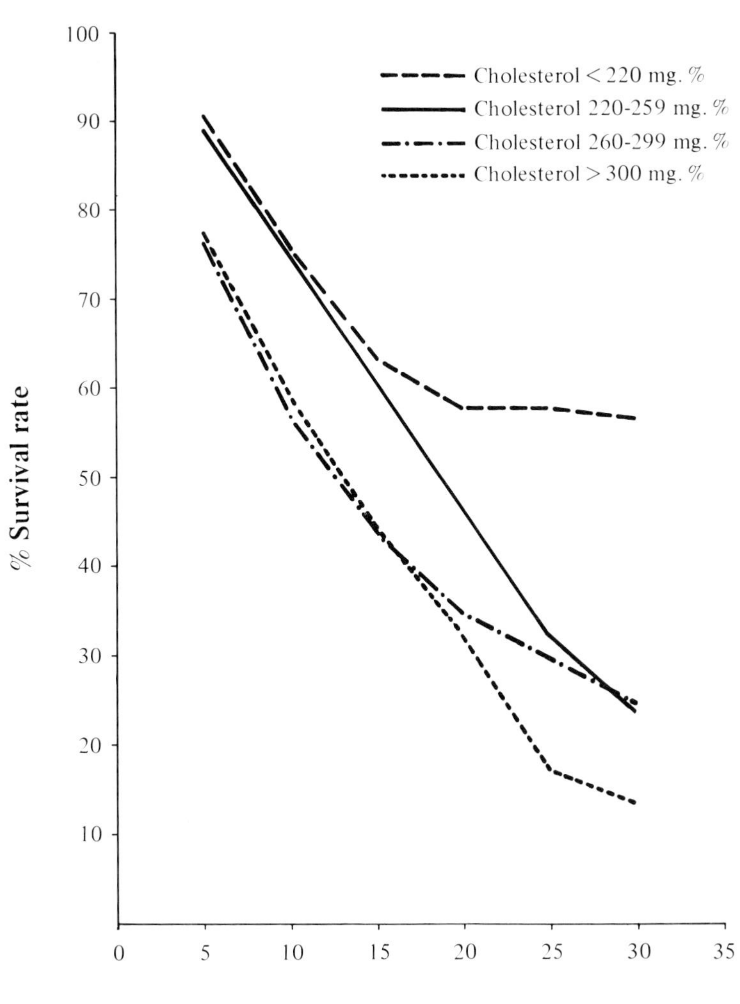

Figure 10.3 Survival rates based on cholesterol above and below 300 mg. %—a three-point moving average

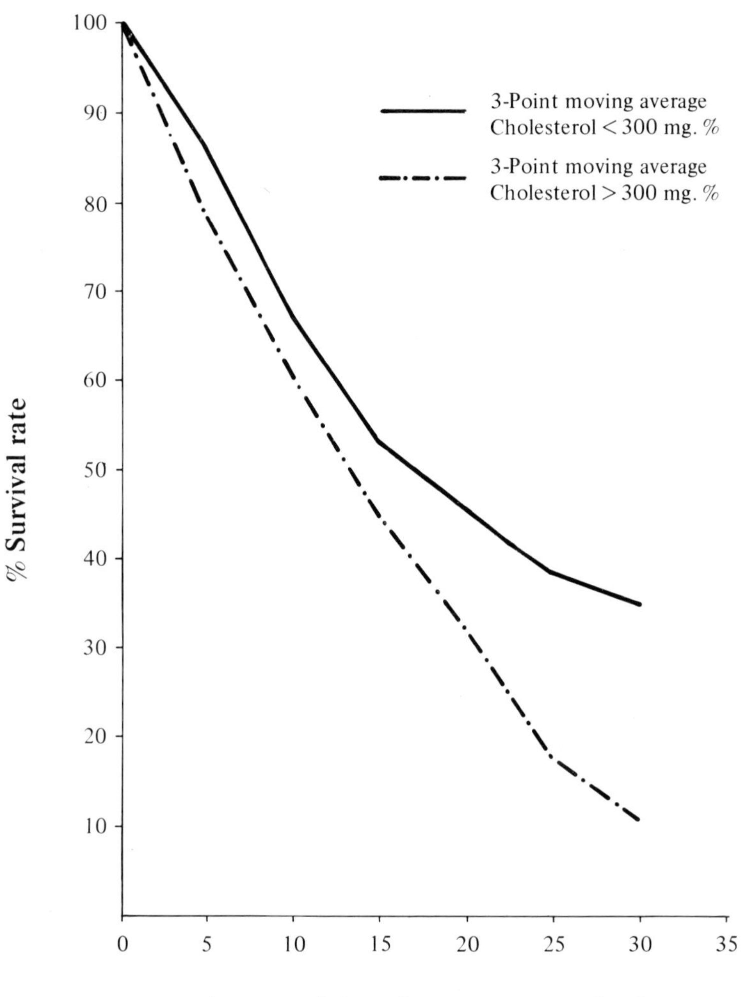

remained at virtually five times the fasting level at three hours postprandial, as compared to the controls whose IRI returned to two times the fasting level. In the coronary heart disease group and the control group, both the glucose tolerance curves and the IRI curves approximated each other at all time intervals (see Table 10.15). The evidence pointed to a vast difference in the serum glucose and IRI responses following an oral G.T.T. in the ITCVD group as compared to the coronary heart disease group. This observation, coupled with the fact that the serum cholesterol limits were significantly higher in the coronary population than in the ITCVD group, pointed to a basic difference between the two groups; namely, the ITCVD group appears to have had a more dominant carbohydrate abnormality, whereas the coronary group had a more dominant lipid abnormality.

This view is reinforced with an analysis of the lactate and free fatty acid responses in the groups during an oral glucose tolerance test.

Free fatty acids (F.F.A.). There is a distinct difference in free fatty acid levels between ischemic heart disease patients with normal oral glucose tolerance tests and those with abnormal glucose tolerance tests. Table 10.16 illustrates this point along with Figure 10.4. While both the control and C.H.D. groups in both the normal and abnormal G.T.T. categories had almost identical values at their nadirs, which occurred at two hours, the C.H.D. group with abnormal glucose tolerance response had a significantly lower rebound level at three hours ($p<.05$) when compared to both control groups.

Lactate levels. In the age-matched control subjects with normal G.T.T.s, the lactate levels reached a sharp peak at one hour, followed by a rapid decline to below fasting level at three hours. The mean lactate curves of the control subjects with abnormal G.T.T.s and C.H.D. patients with normal and abnormal G.T.T.s exhibited lagging maximum lactate levels at one and two hours. The C.H.D. patients with abnormal G.T.T.s had the highest lactate levels at all time intervals, and the fasting, the three-hour lactate, and the sum lactate levels were significantly higher when compared to the control subjects with abnormal G.T.T.s.

Lipoprotein electrophoretic pattern. Chi square analysis revealed a significantly greater frequency ($p<.001$) of abnormal lipoprotein patterns in 45 C.H.D. subjects than in 91 control subjects. It is interesting that in the 77 subjects with normal lipoprotein patterns, 62 had normal and 15 had abnormal G.T.T.s. In the 59 subjects with lipoprotein abnormalities, 37 had normal and 22 had abnormal G.T.T.s. The chi square analysis of the lipoprotein and G.T.T. classification yielded a significant dependence ($p<.05$), which indicated that lipoprotein abnormalities accompany abnormal G.T.T.s. Table 10.17 summarizes the data.

The coefficient correlations and the canonical correlations offer some theoretical explanation for the differences in these data. In the C.H.D. patients, but not in the age-matched control subjects, the serum total cholesterol and lipid phosphorus were significantly and positively correlated with the half- and one-hour glucose levels, and cholesterol was further correlated with the one-hour IRI level. It is reasonable to assume that the elevated half- and one-hour glucose levels contributed in some significant, as yet unknown, manner to the elevated cholesterol and lipid phosphorus levels in C.H.D. patients only. These observations are somewhat similar to those reported by Hatch et

Table 10.9 Comparison of survival rate for first 10 years in coronary group for cholesterol less than 220 mg. % and higher levels

Years survived	<220 mg. %		220-259 mg. %				260-299 mg. %				300-339 mg. %				>340 mg. %			
	No.	Survival rate	No.	Survival rate	t	p<	No.	Survival rate	t	p<	No.	Survival rate	t	p<	No.	Survival rate	t	p<
1	19	1.0	17	1.0	0.0	ns	21	.90	1.11	ns	26	1.0	0.0	ns	15	.93	1.16	ns
2	19	1.0	17	.94	1.0	ns	21	.86	1.75	ns	26	.96	1.00	ns	15	.80	2.0	ns
3	19	1.0	17	.94	1.0	ns	21	.86	1.75	ns	26	.92	1.60	ns	15	.80	2.0	ns
4	19	1.0	17	.94	1.0	ns	21	.81	2.38	.05	26	.85	2.14	.05	15	.80	2.0	ns
5	19	.95	17	.94	0.12	ns	21	.76	1.84	ns	26	.81	1.48	ns	15	.67	2.15	.05
6	19	.95	17	.88	0.70	ns	21	.76	1.84	ns	26	.77	1.91	ns	15	.60	2.50	.05
7	19	.95	17	.88	0.70	ns	21	.76	1.84	ns	26	.73	0.91	ns	15	.60	2.50	.05
8	19	.84	17	.88	0.35	ns	21	.71	1.01	ns	26	.62	1.83	ns	15	.60	1.57	ns
9	19	.79	17	.82	0.28	ns	21	.62	1.26	ns	26	.62	1.33	ns	15	.60	1.20	ns
10	19	.74	17	.71	0.20	ns	21	.57	1.14	ns	26	.62	0.85	ns	15	.60	0.85	ns

Table 10.10 Comparison of long-term survival rates of coronary patients with serum cholesterol less than 220 mg. % to those with higher levels

Years survived	<220 mg. %		220-259 mg. %				260-299 mg. %				300-339 mg. %				>340 mg. %			
	No.	Survival rate	No.	Survival rate	t	p<	No.	Survival rate	t	p<	No.	Survival rate	t	p<	No.	Survival rate	t	p<
20	19	.58	17	.53	0.31	ns	21	.38	1.28	ns	26	.27	2.18	.05	15	.47	0.65	ns
25	19	.58	17	.24	2.28	.05	21	.29	1.95	ns	26	.12	3.67	.01	15	.20	2.55	.05
30	19	.58	17	.24	2.28	.05	21	.24	2.39	.05	26	.08	4.13	.001	15	.13	3.16	.01
35	19	.58	17	.24	1.95	ns	21	.24	2.04	.05	26	.08	3.72	.001	15	.13	3.16	.01

Table 10.11 Differences in survival rates of coronary patients with serum cholesterol above and below 300 mg. %

Years survived	Cholesterol <300 mg. % Number at risk	Survival rate	± S.E.	Cholesterol >300 mg. % Number at risk	Survival rate	± S.E.	t	p<
5	57	0.88	.04	41	0.76	.07	1.71	ns
10	57	0.67	.06	41	0.61	.08	0.64	ns
15	57	0.51	.07	41	0.44	.08	0.70	ns
20	57	0.49	.07	41	0.34	.07	1.69	ns
25	57	0.37	.06	41	0.15	.06	2.86	.01
30	57	0.35	.06	41	0.10	.05	3.57	.001
35	57	0.33	.06	41	0.10	.05	3.29	.01

Table 10.12 Mean and standard error of variables for C.H.D. males and age-matched controls, and ITCVD males and age-matched controls

Variable	C.H.D. males $\bar{X}$	± S.E.	Age-matched controls for C.H.D. $\bar{X}$	± S.E.	ITCVD males $\bar{X}$	± S.E.	Age-matched controls for ITCVD $\bar{X}$	± S.E.
Age	53	1.0	53	1.0	62	1.6	60	1.6
Height	68	0.5	69	0.3	67	0.4	68	0.4
Weight	168	4.5	173	3.2	157	3.1	165	4.3
Systolic B.P.	131	3.2	131	2.7	146	3.9	131	2.8
Diastolic B.P.	81	1.7	82	1.7	84	2.2	80	2.0
Thyroxine μ mg. %	4.7	0.13	4.7	0.12	4.9	0.14	4.7	0.17
Cholesterol mg. %	250	6.8	230	5.8	219	6.6	223	7.7
Lipid phosphorus mg. %	10.4	0.20	9.9	0.23	9.7	0.28	9.8	0.29
Triglycerides mg. %	156	8.7	153	13.8	155	8.5	134	15.3
Uric acid mg. %	6.2	0.18	5.7	0.18	6.1	0.23	5.8	0.26
Sum glucose mg. %	577	13.9	577	12.7	646	25.4	600	14.7
Sum insulin μ U./ml	234	18.8	235	21.6	358	40.8	233	20.6
Total N=168	N=51		N=51		N=33		N=33	

$\bar{X}$ = Mean value
S.E. = Standard error of mean

Reproduced with permission from "Covert Diabetes Mellitus in Ischemic Heart and Cerebrovascular Disease," by Menard M. Gertler, M.D., Hillar E. Leetma, M.D., Erich Saluste, Ph.D., Donald A. Covalt, M.D., and James L. Rosenberger, B.A., *Geriatrics,* Vol. 27, No. 3, pp. 105-116. Copyright The New York Times Media Company, Inc.

Table 10.13 Percentage of abnormal and normal glucose tolerance tests in male C.H.D. patients and matched controls, and male ITCVD patients and matched controls

	C.H.D. males		Matched controls	ITCVD males		Matched controls
Number	51		51	33		33
Normal	57		69	27		46
Abnormal	43		31	73		54
Significance		ns			$p < .01$	
X^2		2.59			6.98	

Table 10.14 Immunoreactive insulin response for C.H.D. males and matched controls, and ITCVD males and matched controls

Time (hours)	C.H.D. males Mean ± S.E.	Matched controls Mean ± S.E.	ITCVD males Mean ± S.E.	Matched controls Mean ± S.E.
Fasting	15.2 ± 0.99	14.8 ± 1.31	16.7 ± 1.69	14.2 ± 1.76
½	46.6 ± 0.35	62.0 ± 6.89	64.9 ± 11.60	57.4 ± 7.22
1	76.3 ± 9.78	76.4 ± 9.17	93.0 ± 15.06	71.5 ± 6.81
2	67.4 ± 6.46	56.4 ± 6.85	106.4 ± 13.99	56.4 ± 6.48
3	28.4 ± 2.82	25.3 ± 2.75	77.5 ± 6.85	33.8 ± 5.84
Sum	234	235	358	233
S.E.	18.8	21.6	40.8	20.6

al.,[5] and Heinle et al.[6] In the control group, the triglycerides were more strongly correlated with the glucose and IRI levels than in the C.H.D. group. This may be related to the somewhat delayed and elevated IRI response in C.H.D. patients.

The three strongest canonical correlations—found between IRI and glucose, IRI and F.F.A., and IRI and lactate levels—imply that insulin is the controlling factor in both carbohydrate and lipid metabolism. It is possible that prolonged and excessive availability of insulin promotes conversion of more glucose to F.F.A. and also the trapping of more F.F.A. in tissues as triglycerides, phospholipids, and cholesterol.

The elevated uric acid levels found in subjects with abnormal G.T.T.s are significant since it has been postulated by Galzigna et al. that uric acid is a potent inhibitor of monoamine oxidase.[7] Cegrell et al. have theorized that the inhibition of monoamine oxidase could affect the biogenic amine levels in the pancreatic beta cells and thereby effect increased insulin secretion.[8]

A possible explanation for the accumulation of lactate in C.H.D. patients with abnormal G.T.T.s is the excessive availability of F.F.A. and competition for the availability of coenzyme A for the decarboxylation of pyruvate (see Figure 10.4), which supports the existence of a glucose-F.F.A. cycle as suggested by Randle, Hales et al.[9]

The evidence suggests that the current view that diabetes mellitus is an important

Table 10.15 Glucose tolerance test responses for C.H.D. males and matched controls, and ITCVD males and matched controls

Time (hours)	C.H.D. males Mean ± S.E.	Matched controls Mean ± S.E.	ITCVD males Mean ± S.E.	Matched controls Mean ± S.E.
Fasting	95 ± 1.9	94 ± 1.3	92 ± 2.5	96 ± 2.1
½	141 ± 3.1	153 ± 3.3	134 ± 4.0	153 ± 4.5
1	146 ± 5.3	145 ± 5.9	159 ± 7.5	154 ± 6.5
2	112 ± 4.5	108 ± 4.6	144 ± 7.5	114 ± 5.9
3	84 ± 3.5	78 ± 7.3	117 ± 8.3	85 ± 4.3
Sum	578	578	646	602
S.E.	13.9	12.7	25.4	14.7

Table 10.16 Mean free fatty acid levels in C.H.D. males and control subjects aged 45-64 years, with abnormal and normal glucose tolerance response

	Normal G.T.T.		Abnormal G.T.T.	
	Controls (n=33)	C.H.D. (n=22)	Controls (n=10)	C.H.D. (n=17)
Fasting	426	374	434	472
½	346	334	333	379
1	222	208	235	255
2	180	157	129	156
3	274	191	254	175

risk factor in coronary heart disease should be altered somewhat.[10] There are considerable overlappings of and interrelationships between both carbohydrate and lipid metabolism in both coronary heart disease and ischemic thrombotic cerebrovascular disease. The major interpretative difference is one of emphasis. Diabetes mellitus and carbohydrate metabolic abnormalities exist to a predominant extent in cerebrovascular disease, whereas lipid abnormalities are more predominant in coronary heart disease. We urge our colleagues to recognize that the one- or two-hour glucose levels after a glucose load give only limited and screening information and do not begin to have the value of a complete glucose tolerance test, which studies other aspects of lipid and carbohydrate interrelationships. A related factor is the relationship of uric acid abnormalities to carbohydrate and triglyceride abnormalities, which has been discussed in Chapter VII.

Psychological factors

The assessment of personality types in the study of coronary heart disease has intrigued many investigators. Sheldon reviewed the historical contribution to this subject,[11] but it remained for Dunbar to implicate a definite personality type in C.H.D.[12] A more sophisticated investigation was massed by Rosenman, Friedman, and Strauss, who described a behavioral type considered characteristic of the coronary-prone individual.[13]

Table 10.17 Lipoprotein electrophoretic patterns in male C.H.D. and control subjects

Group	G.T.T.	Type II	Type IV	Normal	Total
C.H.D.	Normal	1	14	9	24 (53%)
	Abnormal	1	15	5	21 (47%)
	Total	2 (4%)	29 (65%)	14 (31%)	45 (100%)
Control	Normal	2	20	53	75 (82%)
	Abnormal	0	6	10	16 (18%)
	Total	2 (2%)	26 (29%)	63 (69%)	91 (100%)

Permission to reproduce granted by The American Heart Association, Inc. and M. M. Gertler, H. E. Leetma, E. Saluste et al., "Ischemic Heart Disease: Insulin, Carbohydrate, and Lipid Interrelationships," *Circulation* 46: 103-111, 1972.

These individuals, known as Type A, were found to have six times the incidence of coronary heart disease as Type B individuals. Type A individuals are characterized by overambition, high drive, and constant time-stress behavior. Type B individuals do not display these personality characteristics.

A psychological appraisal was undertaken by Gordon et al., on patients who had recovered from coronary heart disease and control subjects.[14] The group of control subjects consisted of low- and high-profile-score individuals. The assessment of profile scores was based on the methods described in the present study. The average ages of the patients and control subjects were virtually the same, that is, 54.5±9.0 years in the coronary group and 46.9±14.9 and 49.8±12.0 years in the low- and high-profile controls, respectively. The study was executed in a double blind manner.

The psychological appraisal was obtained through the use of three tests: (a) Zuckerman Multiple Affect Adjective Checklist,[15] (b) People Test,[16] and (c) the 42-item Q-sort developed by Gordon and Diller and based on the work of Jenkins, Zyzanski, Rosenman,[17] and Bortner.[18] The Zuckerman Multiple Affect Adjective Checklist is scored in standard fashion for anxiety, hostility, and depression. The People Test is one in which the subject is asked to name all the people he came in contact with or thought about the day before. The responses are scored for content (number of family members named, number of work people named). The particular Q-sort used here consisted of seven positive and seven negative items representing each of the three aspects of behavior relevant to coronary-prone status. These three domains were: impatience/speed (I eat rapidly; I am a good listener), job involvement (I bring office work home with me; I relax during my lunch hour), and hard driving (I like to win; I am a relaxed person). This task was administered according to procedures outlined by Stephenson.[19]

The coronary heart disease group had a significantly higher score ($p<.05$) on all three Zuckerman scales (anxiety, hostility, and depression) than either of the two control groups. There appeared to be little difference between the two control groups. However, the high-risk healthy group gave more socially desirable responses. An interesting finding was that both the high-risk group and the low-risk group could be distinguished from each other as could the C.H.D. and low-risk groups in the adjective self-assessment phase of the

Figure 10.4 Mean F.F.A. response curves in male C.H.D. and control subjects (age range 45-64 years) according to normal and abnormal G.T.T.

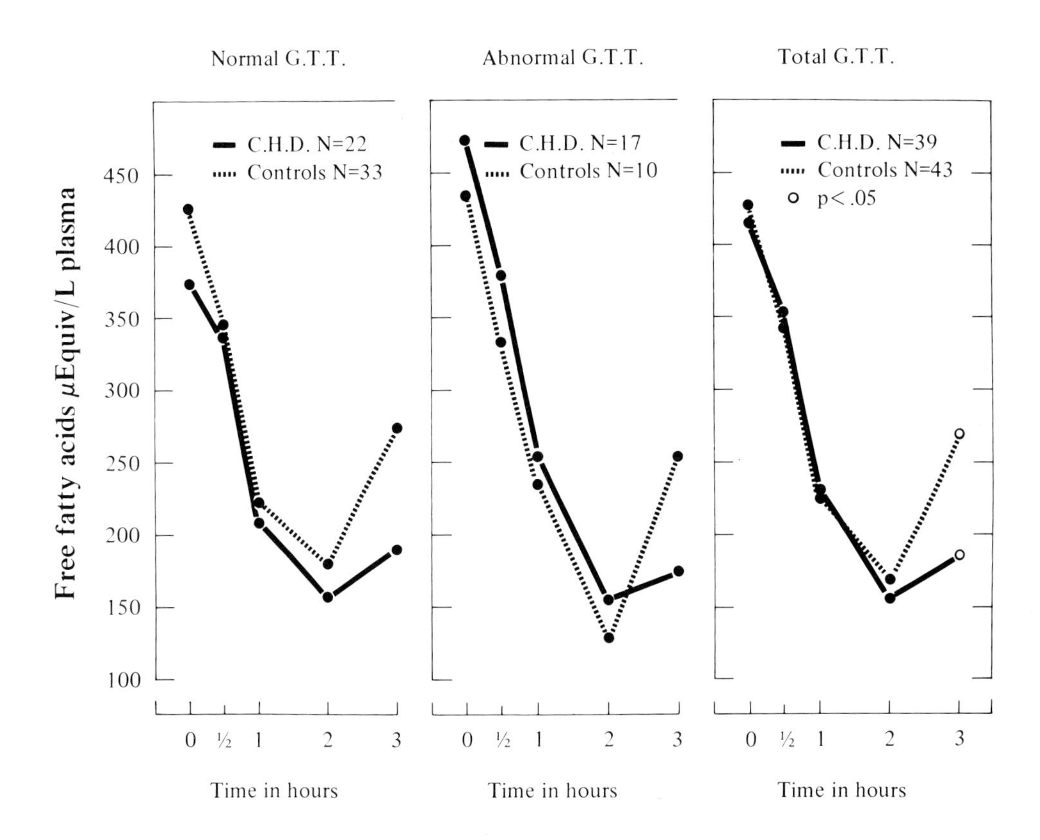

Permission to reproduce granted by The American Heart Association, Inc. and M. M. Gertler, H. E. Leetma, E. Saluste et al., "Ischemic Heart Disease: Insulin, Carbohydrate, and Lipid Interrelationships," *Circulation* 46: 103-111, 1972.

test ($p<.05$), called the positive self-presentation ratio. However, the C.H.D. and high-risk groups could not be distinguished from each other. This latter finding indicated a basic problem that will not be solved until members of the high-risk group experience an acute event and then are retested. Perhaps the tendency to overpresent oneself will manifest itself more under these conditions.

The People Test recorded equal performance in all three study groups for naming the actual number of people. However, the differentiation manifested itself in the choice of names. For example, the low- and high-risk groups associated two or more family-peer names and six or fewer work-associated names; the C.H.D. group associated fewer than two family names and more than seven work-related names. Thus it may be inferred that the C.H.D. individual is work-oriented—an indication of competitiveness, time urgency, and an inability to relax, all of which have been associated with heart disease.[20]

The Q-sort did not reveal any significant differences. However, there were certain interesting trends; for example, the low-risk group tended to cluster in the job involvement scale, whereas the high-risk group clustered in the impatience and speed scales.

We explored the possibility of assembling all the psychological responses to obtain a better discrimination between the groups than single tests could provide. The scores for the high- and low-risk subjects were replaced with appropriate plus and minus signs and then summed. A summary score table was presented that, in effect, was able to distinguish between the two groups ($p<.001$). This analysis resulted in the correct classification of 92 per cent (23 of 25 subjects) of the "healthy" individuals.

This study emphasized the possibility of distinguishing high- and low-prone individuals to C.H.D. by psychological assessment. It appears that coronary proneness is not represented in an "either/or" personality type but rather by various differences over a constellation of factors.

The Terman Miles test was given to the original coronary and control groups to determine to what extent these individuals fitted the typically masculine or feminine patterns of our culture.[21] It was hoped that some clues would be revealed as to whether the characteristics usually associated with psychological masculinity or femininity influence the susceptibility of the individual to coronary heart disease.

The coronary group scored significantly lower (15 points lower) on the average than did the matched control group for all seven exercises of the test. The test revealed that the coronary heart disease patients, as a group, were somewhat less aggressive, less adventurous, less enterprising, and less self-assertive than the control group. They were actively sympathetic and concerned with domestic affairs, art, and literature.

These results may be surprising in view of the fact that many of the coronary patients have been described as hard-driving and determined to succeed. The apparent contradiction, however, has several possible explanations. The very fact that these men were able to push through to success in their enterprises may well have put them in a position to participate increasingly in the more cultural aspects of our society, thereby modifying their interests and attitudes in the direction considered more typically feminine. Furthermore, at the time of testing, most of the patients had experienced some degree of invalidism, which in itself may have led to the adoption of more sympathetic attitudes and more sedentary and intellectual interests.

One may seriously question whether the characteristics usually associated with psychological masculinity or femininity influence the susceptibility of the individual to coronary heart disease. Even though we have found that the typical patient originally showed masculine traits that were later modified toward femininity, can we assume that, in general, overt characteristics of masculinity in a healthy male are indicative of covert characteristics that may enhance susceptibility to coronary heart disease? And, conversely, if a healthy male shows overt feminine characteristics, can we assume that these are indicative of covert characteristics that confer protection against the disease? Hamilton avoids "the often tempting, but naive, tendency to ascribe all conditions associated with one sex solely to the temperaments, habits, or environment of the members of that sex."[22] However, whether or not such characteristics as aggressiveness, boldness, and love of adventure can causally relate to coronary heart disease, they may possibly express some hormonal factor linked closely to the etiology of C.H.D.

Cigarette smoking

The statistical evidence appears to be overwhelmingly that cigarette smoking is associated not only with increased mortality from coronary heart disease[23] but also increased risk of stroke and occlusive peripheral vascular disease.[24] The evidence continues to implicate such diseases as cancer of the mouth, larynx, pharynx, and lungs as well. In addition to these diseases, evidence appears to indicate that physical fitness and endurance are compromised in the cigarette smoker,[25] and that cessation of smoking produces a reversal of the malevolent effects attributed to smoking.[26]

Statistical associative evidence is, of course, subject to reinterpretation and re-evaluation. There is, however, additional finite evidence indicating that smoking produces an increased binding of acridine in epithelial cells, out of proportion to the DNA content.[27] There are also data showing that cigarette smoking is proportional to blood carboxyhemoglobin levels (CoHb), which have a direct relationship to atherosclerotic diseases.[28] The evidence appears one-sided and overwhelming, though there are a few inconsistencies in the evidence.

Seltzer has accumulated evidence supporting the view that cigarette smokers and coronary heart disease patients share the same constitutional or body type.[29] He points out certain inconsistencies in the results of studies on the cigarette-coronary heart disease association: (a) The relationship between daily cigarette inhalation and duration of cigarette smoking does not produce a linear relationship between these variables and mortality and/or morbidity, and (b) the pathologic reports do not show any correlation between antecedent premorbid cigarette smoking and degree of uncomplicated coronary atherosclerosis.

Such evidence must be taken into consideration when determining and evaluating the role of cigarette smoking as a risk factor in coronary heart disease.

Ischemic Thrombotic Cerebrovascular Disease

A direct outgrowth of the development of a profile score to identify those individuals prone to coronary heart disease was the development of a profile score for the identification of individuals incubating ischemic thrombotic cerebrovascular disease.[30]

The high incidence of ITCVD, particularly in the elderly, has made early recognition and prevention of this disease of paramount importance. In the age group 60-70 years, about three individuals per 1,000–both men and women–experience ITCVD each year. However, the long incubation period of ITCVD makes it possible to recognize this disease during its covert stage and institute primary preventive therapy to delay and/or forestall the overt event. Since C.H.D. and ITCVD are both atherothrombotic and possess some

Figure 10.5 Schematic representation of individual risk factors for the classification of C.H.D. (I.H.D.)- and ITCVD-prone individuals

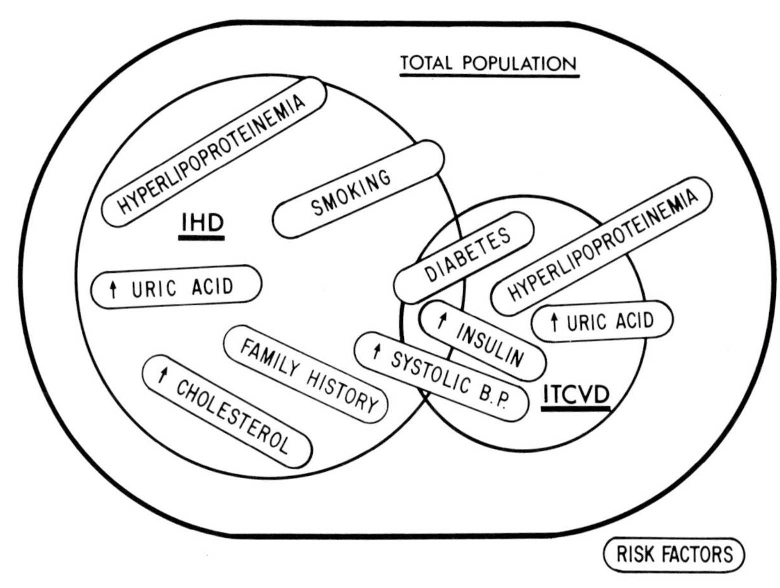

Permission to reproduce granted by The American Heart Association, Inc. and M. M. Gertler, J. L. Rosenberger, and H. E. Leetma, "Identification of Individuals With Covert Ischemic Thrombotic Cerebrovascular Disease: A Discriminant Function Analysis," *Stroke* 3: 764-771, 1972.

risk factors in common (see Figure 10.5), it is reasonable to extend similar techniques to the identification of individuals prone to ITCVD.

The following biochemical tests were made on venous blood in a group of ITCVD and control subjects: fasting serum cholesterol, lipid phosphorus, triglycerides, uric acid, and lipoprotein electrophoretic patterns. A three-hour oral glucose tolerance was administered to the diseased group and healthy age-matched controls. Blood glucose, immunoreactive insulin, and free fatty acid levels were determined on fasting and following the ingestion of the equivalent of 75 grams of glucose in the form of Glucola, at half-, one-, two-, and three-hour intervals. Clinical measurements included blood pressure, height, weight, ponderal index, electrocardiogram, chest X-ray, complete blood count, blood urea nitrogen, electrolytes, thyroxine, and liver profile.

The continuous variables, such as cholesterol and uric acid, were individually compared between the ITCVD group and the age-matched control group for a difference in the mean, using a two-tailed t-test where applicable. The categorical variables, such as presence or absence of hypertension, normal or abnormal electrocardiogram (ECG), and lipoprotein patterns, were tested for discriminating power with a chi square analysis. All study variables showing differences between the two groups were considered risk factors of ITCVD and were included in the multivariate discriminant analysis. In cases where one or more data items were missing, the grand mean of the variable was inserted for the missing data.

No significant differences were found in height, weight, ponderal index, cholesterol, and lipid phosphorus levels between the disease and control group.

The discriminant function analysis of the risk factors was accomplished in a stepwise manner, that is, at each step of the analysis all the variables not yet entered into the function were tested to select the next most discriminating variable. In addition, the F ratio was calculated and tested to ensure that each risk factor in the function contributed significantly to the discrimination between the disease and healthy groups. The stepwise procedure was terminated when the remaining variables provided no additional contribution to the over-all discrimination.

Significantly elevated systolic and diastolic blood pressures; elevated glucose, triglyceride, and uric acid levels; abnormal IRI, F.F.A., and lactate response in ITCVD indicated that any one of these variables can be considered as an individual risk factor and may be predictive of ITCVD. Chi square analyses of lipoprotein patterns, history of hypertension, and electrocardiograms revealed a significantly greater prevalence of these abnormalities in ITCVD than in control subjects.

Table 10.18 introduces the results obtained for this discriminant function analysis. The function coefficients represent each variable in its natural units and for this reason cannot be used as an absolute measure of discriminating power. However, weighting the function coefficients of each variable with their standard deviation results in a new coefficient not dependent on any unit measure.

In the standardized coefficients of the primary risk factors of ITCVD, the IRI three-hour level was the most powerful individual discriminator, followed by an abnormal lipoprotein pattern, G.T.T. two-hour level, and systolic blood pressure. In using zero as the best criterion for discriminating between the ITCVD and age-matched control subjects, the discriminant function with these four primary risk factors resulted in correct classification of 84.4 per cent of these subjects.

The application of the discriminant function in an actual screening program is demonstrated by the following example. A positive profile score indicates proneness to ITCVD, a negative score nonproneness.

	Nonprone subject	Prone subject
IRI three-hour level (μ units/ml)	47	28
Lipoprotein pattern	Normal	Abnormal
G.T.T. two-hour level (mg. %)	91	110
Systolic B.P. (mm Hg)	120	168
Profile score	–1.48	+1.34

The entire set of variables in Table 10.18 (with the addition of ECG, which shows a significant difference) can be considered as risk factors of ITCVD. Variables such as diastolic blood pressure, uric acid, triglycerides, F.F.A. and lactate three-hour levels, and ECG abnormalities demonstrate univariate discriminating power. But when each is included in the multivariate function as an additional variable to the set of more powerful discriminators, its additional contribution to the classification of ITCVD-prone individuals is not significant. However, it must be remembered that each of these variables may be considered clinically as an indicator of covert ITCVD.

Table 10.18 Discriminant function of the primary risk factors of ITCVD

Variable (X_i)	Function coefficient (C_i)	S.D.	Standardized coefficient
IRI 3-hour level (μ units/ml)	0.033	(42.2)	1.40
Systolic B.P. (mm Hg)	0.039	(21.1)	0.83
Lipoprotein (1,2)*	2.480	(0.502)	1.24
Glucose 2-hour level (mg. %)	0.020	(45.4)	0.91
Constant (C_o)	−13.300		

*Code: 1-normal, 2-abnormal

Discriminant function score: $Y = \sum_i C_i X_i + C_o$ = 0.033 x (IRI 3 hours) + 0.039 x (systolic B.P.) + 2.48 x (lipoprotein) + 0.020 x (glucose 2 hours) −13.3

Permission to reproduce granted by The American Heart Association, Inc. and M. M. Gertler, J. L. Rosenberger, and H. E. Leetma, "Identification of Individuals With Covert Ischemic Thrombotic Cerebrovascular Disease: A Discriminant Function Analysis," *Stroke* 3: 764-771, 1972.

The discriminant function calculated for the ITCVD profile was generated from a retrospective study, as was the C.H.D. profile. A prospective study is in progress to determine the degree of validity of this equation in early recognition.

Summary

The modern epidemic of coronary heart disease lends itself to preventive measures by virtue of its long incubation period. In contradistinction, the acute infectious diseases have a short incubation period (two to three weeks) which makes preventive and curative methods almost superimposable and of dire necessity. While enabling one to institute early preventive therapy, the long incubation period is also a handicap because of the absence of symptomatology. In addition, the usual statement of neurotic indifference ("It is only statistical and it probably will not affect me") becomes part of the lexicon.

Early recognition and early prevention of coronary heart disease, the importance of which was recognized by Gertler, Garn, and White in 1951,[31] has now become an official National Institute of Health Program in the form of the Multiple Risk Factor Intervention Trial for the Prevention of Coronary Heart Disease. The results of this vast undertaking will be of importance not only to Americans but to people throughout the world.

As yet, unanimity is lacking on the question of which risk factors should be used to discriminate the highest number of candidates for the disease. This matter will be resolved eventually; in the meantime, small differences of opinion should not be permitted to stand in the way of salvaging the lives of hundreds of thousands of men and women by at least delaying the onset of C.H.D. and perhaps preventing the disease altogether.

References

1 S. A. Levine, "Angina Pectoris: Some Clinical Considerations," *JAMA* 79: 928-937, 1922; E. P. Joslin, "Arteriosclerosis and Diabetes," *Ann. Clin. Med.* 5: 1061-1080, 1927.

2 G. Cabrera and M. M. Gertler, "Enzymatic and Hormonal Control of Fatty Acid Synthesis," *Circulation* 16: 486-487, 1957.

3 M. J. Albrink and P. C. Davidson, "Impaired Glucose Tolerance in Patients With Hypertriglyceridemia," *J. Lab. Clin. Med.* 67: 573-584, 1966; W. R. Harlan Jr., A. Oberman, R. E. Mitchell, and A. Graybel, "Constitutional and Environmental Factors Related to Serum Lipid and Lipoprotein Levels," *Ann. Int. Med.* 66: 540-555, 1967.

4 M. M. Gertler, H. E. Leetma, E. Saluste et al., "Ischemic Heart Disease: Insulin, Carbohydrate and Lipid Interrelationships," *Circulation* 46: 103-111, 1972; M. M. Gertler, H. E. Leetma, E. Saluste et al., "Covert Diabetes Mellitus in Ischemic Heart and Cerebrovascular Disease," *Geriatrics* 27: 105-116, 1972.

5 F. T. Hatch, P. K. Reissel, T. M. W. Pook-King et al., "A Study of Coronary Heart Disease in Young Men: Characteristics and Metabolic Studies of the Patients and Comparison With Age-Matched Healthy Men," *Circulation* 33: 679-703, 1966.

6 R. A. Heinle, R. I. Levy, and D. S. Fredrickson, "Lipid and Carbohydrate Abnormalities in Patients With Angiographically Documented Coronary Artery Disease," *Amer. J. Cardiol.* 24: 178-186, 1969.

7 L. Galzigna, G. Maina, and G. Rumney, "Role of L-Ascorbic Acid in the Reversal of the Monoamine Oxidase Inhibition by Caffeine," *J. Pharm. Pharmacol.* 23: 303-305, 1971.

8 L. Cegrell, B. Falk, and B. Hellman, "Monoaminergic Mechanisms in the Endocrine Pancreas," in *The Structure and Metabolism of the Pancreatic Islets,* S. E. Brolin, B. Hellman, H. Knutson, eds. (New York: Macmillan Co., 1964), p. 429.

9 P. J. Randle, C. N. Hales, P. B. Garland, and E. A. Newsholme, "The Glucose Fatty-Acid Cycle: Its Role in Insulin-Sensitivity and the Metabolic Disturbances of Diabetes Mellitus," *Lancet* 1: 785-794, 1963.

10 F. E. Epstein, "Hyperglycemia," *Circulation* 36: 609-619, 1967; W. B. Kannel and T. Gordon, eds., *The Framingham Study: An Epidemiological Investigation of Cardiovascular Disease,* Section 27, (Washington, D.C.: U.S. Government Printing Office, May 1971), p. 9; J. Stamler, D. M. Berkson, and H. A. Lindberg, "Risk Factors: Their Role in the Etiology and Pathogenesis of the Atherosclerotic Diseases," in *The Pathogenesis of Atherosclerosis,* R. W. Wissler and J. C. Geer, eds. (Baltimore: Williams and Wilkins Co., 1972), pp. 41-119.

11 W. H. Sheldon, S. S. Stevens, and W. B. Tucker, *The Varieties of Human Physique* (New York: Harper and Bros., 1940), pp. 300-310.

12 F. Dunbar, *Psychosomatic Diagnosis* (New York: Hoeber, 1943), pp. 248-365.

13 R. H. Rosenman, M. Friedman, R. Strauss et al., "Coronary Heart Abuses in the Western Collaborative Group Study," *JAMA* 198: 15-22, 1966.

14 W. A. Gordon, M. M. Gertler, L. Diller, H. Leetma, L. Gerstman, "Behavioral Correlates of the Coronary Profile," *J. Clin. Psych.* 343-347, July, 1974.

15 M. Zuckerman and B. Lubin, *Multiple Affect Adjective Checklist* (San Diego: Educational and Industrial Testing Service, 1965).

16 L. Diller, W. Gordon, C. Swinyard, and S. Kastner, "Psychological and Educational Studies With Spina Bifida Children," *Final Report, Proj. No.* 5-0412, OEG 32-42-8145-5020 (Washington, D.C.: U.S. Office of Education, 1964), pp. 1-130.

17 C. D. Jenkins, S. S. Zyzanski, R. H. Rosenman et al., "Recent Developments in Defining and Measuring Behavioral Risk Factors in Coronary Heart Disease," *Psychosom. Med.* 31: 446, 1969.

18 R. W. Bortner, "A Short Rating Scale as a Potential Measure of Pattern A Behavior," *J. Chron. Dis.* 22: 87-91, 1966.

19 W. Stephenson, *The Study of Behavior* (Chicago: University of Chicago Press, 1953), pp. 1-376.

20 J. Bastiaans, "Psychoanalytic Investigations on the Psychic Aspects of Acute Myocardial Infarction," *Psychother. Psychosom.* 16: 202-209, 1968; C. D. Jenkins, "Psychologic and Social Precursors of Coronary Disease," *New Eng. J. Med.* 284: 244-255, 307-317, 1971; Rosenman et al., "Coronary Heart Abuses," pp. 15-22.

21 L. M. Terman and C. C. Miles, *Sex and Personality* (New York: McGraw-Hill, 1936), pp. 1-600.

22 J. B. Hamilton, "The Role of Testicular Secretions as Indicated by the Effects of Castration in Men and by Studies of Pathological Conditions and the Short Life-Span Associated With Maleness," *Recent Prog. in Hormone Research* 3: 257-322, 1948.

23 U.S. Public Health Service, "Atherosclerosis," *Health Consequences of Smoking,*

1969 Suppl. (Washington, D.C.: U.S. Government Printing Office, 1969), pp. 25-27.

24 Kannel, *The Framingham Study*, p. 9.

25 K. H. Cooper, G. O. Gey, and R. A. Bottenberg, "Effects of Cigarette Smoking on Endurance Performance," *JAMA* 203: 189-192, 1968; K. H. David, "Age, Cigarette Smoking, and Tests of Physical Fitness," *J. Appl. Psychol.* 52: 296-298, 1968.

26 R. Doll and A. B. Hill, "Mortality in Relation to Smoking: Ten Years' Observations of British Doctors," *Brit. Med. J.* 1(2): 1399-1410, 1964.

27 D. Roth, A. Oppenheim, and D. T. Fredrickson, "DNA-Dependent Dye Binding by Oral Epithelium," *Arch. Environ. Health* 17: 59-61, 1968.

28 P. Astrup et al., "The Effect of Tobacco Smoking on the Dissociation Curve of Oxyhemoglobin," *Scand. J. Clin. Lab. Invest.* 18: 450-457, 1966; S. M. Ayres et al., "Systemic and Myocardial Hemodynamic Responses to Relatively Small Concentrations of Carboxyhemoglobin (CoHb)," *Arch. Environ. Health* 18: 699-709, 1969.

29 C. Seltzer, "Morphologic Constitution and Smoking," *JAMA* 183: 639-645, 1963; C. Seltzer, "The Effect of Cigarette Smoking on Coronary Heart Disease," *Arch. Environ. Health* 20: 418-423, 1970.

30 M. M. Gertler, J. L. Rosenberger, and H. E. Leetma, "Identification of Individuals With Covert Ischemic Thrombotic Cerebrovascular Disease: A Discriminant Function Analysis," *Stroke* 3: 764-771, 1972.

31 M. M. Gertler, S. M. Garn, and P. D. White, "Young Candidates for Coronary Heart Disease," *JAMA* 147: 621-625, 1951.

Appendix

We wish to express our thanks to the many physicians who examined the control and coronary subjects and reported their results in a form suitable for computer analysis.

Charles Aronsohn, M.D.–Paterson, N.J.
Walter F. Barnes, M.D.–South Westport, Mass.
William M. I. Barrett, M.D.–Hartboro, Pa.
John T. Berry, M.D.–North Randolph, Mass.
Nelson Bigelow, M.D.–Landgrove, Vt.
William A. Blodgett, M.D.–Louisville, Ky.
Clifford Boyle, M.D.–Worcester, Mass.
Edward Budnitz, M.D.–Worcester, Mass.
George Bullwinkel, M.D.–Rye, N.Y.
O. Sherman Carlson, M.D.–Corpus Christi, Tex.
Wallace Chin, M.D.–Covina, Calif.
William Clarke, M.D.–Tuckahoe, N.Y.
Marshall Clinton, M.D.–Buffalo, N.Y.
F. V. Corsini, M.D.–Quincy, Mass.
William W. Cox, M.D.–Daytona Beach, Fla.
Timothy Crane, M.D.–Cambridge, Mass.
Benjamin de Guzman, M.D.–Glen Burnie, Mass.
William A. Dowd, M.D.–Arlington, Mass.
Adelaide R. Draper, M.D.–Dorchester, Mass.
Theodore J. Edlich Jr., M.D.–New York, N.Y.
William Egan, M.D.–Boston, Mass.
Stanley J. Evans, M.D.–Bangor, Me.
Edward Feeley, M.D.–Arlington, Mass.
Safety R. First, M.D.–Tulsa, Okla.
Alexander N. Fisher, M.D.–Westwood, Mass.
William H. Floyd, M.D.–Ridgewood, N.J.
George Fontaine, M.D.–Cathom, Mass.
Joseph Franklin, M.D.–Boston, Mass.
Thomas J. Gill, M.D.–Winchester, Mass.
Robert R. Gillespy Jr., M.D.–Jacksonville, Fla.
Isadore Gittelsohn, M.D.–River Edge, N.J.
Henry Gloetzner, M.D.–Norwalk, Conn.
Warren Goorno, M.D.–Concord, Mass.
Jack Gordon, M.D.–San Francisco, Calif.
Morris Gorfine, M.D.–Cambridge, Mass.
George Gregorie, M.D.–Winthrop, Mass.
John W. Handwerker, M.D.–Key Biscayne, Fla.
Peter Hanlon, M.D.–Ridgewood, N.J.
Edward E. Harnagle, M.D.–Los Angeles, Calif.
Gerard Helden, M.D.–Hackensack, N.J.
Enrique A. Herrera, M.D.–Baltimore, Md.
Edward E. Hitt, M.D.–Dallas, Tex.
Alvin Hoffman, M.D.–Tork, Me.
John Tilden Howard, M.D.–Baltimore, Md.
Cornelius F. Ivory, M.D.–Ridgewood, N.J.
Fred Jackson, M.D.–Lynn, Mass.
Raymond O. Johnson, M.D.–Marshfield, Mass.
Gustav Kauffman, M.D.–Winchester, Mass.
Paul Keleher, M.D.–Woburn, Mass.
Francis D. Kenney, M.D.–Munster, Ind.
Herbert A. King, M.D.–Daytona Beach, Fla.
William L. Kraus, M.D.–Dallas, Tex.
Joseph H. LaCasca, M.D.–Ellsworth, Me.
Jacob Lerman, M.D.–Boston, Mass.
Orrin Levin, M.D.–Cambridge, Mass.
Charles R. Lewis, M.D.–St. Louis, Mo.
Charles Liberman, M.D.–Winthrop, Mass.
Samuel N. Lipsett, M.D.–Paramus, N.J.
Rank London, M.D.–Knoxville, Tenn.
C. Rogers Lord, M.D.–Bedford, Mass.
Brock Lynch, M.D.–Malden, Mass.
George MacDonald, M.D.–Boston, Mass.
Allan J. McCarthy, M.D.–Arlington, Mass.
Francis E. McDonough, M.D.–Boston, Mass.
Lawrence W. McGrath, M.D.–Roxbury, Mass.
Joseph H. McSweeny, M.D.–Somerville, Mass.
James J. Macklin Jr., M.D.–Cambridge, Mass.
Francis J. Maguire, M.D.–Waban, Mass.
John P. Malec, M.D.–Madison, Wis.
Clarence C. Maloof, M.D.–Boston, Mass.
Walter Martin, M.D.–Westminster, Calif.
Peter Minch Jr., M.D.–Saddle River, N.J.
Merton Minter, M.D.–San Antonio, Tex.
David Mintz, M.D.–Burlington, Vt.
R. F. Montgomery, M.D.–Garden Grove, Calif.
Albert S. Murphy, M.D.–Boston, Mass.
S. Nacchia, M.D.–Belmont, Mass.
Dennis Natoli, M.D.–River Edge, N.J.
N.W. Nemiroff, M.D.–Oradell, N.J.
David O'Brien, M.D.–Somerville, Mass.
John Ohler, M.D.–New London, N.H.
Edward Anthony Oppenheimer, M.D.–Panorama City, Calif.
Edward Owen, M.D.–Lakeland, Calif.
David Parsons, M.D.–Wayland, Mass.
Anna W. Perkins, M.D.–Westerlo, N.Y.
Carey Peters, M.D.–Boston, Mass.
John H. Poczabut, M.D.–Stamford, Conn.
William Cyrus Pomeroy, M.D.–Los Angeles, Calif.
John Poutas, M.D.–Old Greenwich, Conn.
John Z. Preston, M.D.–Tyron, N.C.
R. Purcell, M.D.–Griffith, Ind.
Arthur Rappeport, M.D.–Quincy, Mass.
James P. Rhoads, M.D.–Wichita, Kan.
Charles D. Roberts, M.D.–Englewood Cliffs, N.J.
H. Rummerman, M.D.–Belmont, Mass.
Kenneth Russel, M.D.–Gray, Me.
B. Russman, M.D.–Somerville, Mass.
Julius Sachs, M.D.–Hartford, Conn.

Nicholas L. Santacross, M.D.–Quincy, Mass.
Sidney Scherlis, M.D.–Baltimore, Md.
Robert S. Schwab, M.D.–Boston, Mass.
Larry G. Seidl, M.D.–Wareham, Mass.
Samuel B. Shuman, M.D.–Dorchester, Mass.
Martin Silbersweig, M.D.–Tenafly, N.J.
Robert Sommer, M.D.–Norwell, Mass.
Hamilton Southworth, M.D.–New York, N.Y.
John Spaulding, M.D.–Melrose, Mass.
Harry F. Stafford, M.D.–Whittier, Calif.
James P. Stanton, M.D.–Norwood, Mass.
Stanley Steinberg, M.D.–Canoga Park, Calif.
Frederick H. Summers, M.D.–Whittier, Calif.
L. Titelbaum, M.D.–Arlington, Mass.
Edward J. Toomey, M.D.–Concord, Mass.
Eugene Tyrell, M.D.–Quincy, Mass.
Lee Underwood, M.D.–Canton, Ohio
William Vikers, M.D.–Buffalo, N.Y.
Robert M. Viola, M.D.–Flushing, N.Y.
Andrew D. Vorr, M.D.–Canton, Mass.
C. Weed, M.D.–Stamford, Conn.
Edward Welch, M.D.–Brookline, Mass.
Milton Wiener, M.D.–Hackensack, N.J.
Myron Wright, M.D.–New York, N.Y.
Albert Young, M.D.–Lexington, Mass.
Sidney Zeitler, M.D.–Malden, Mass.

Index

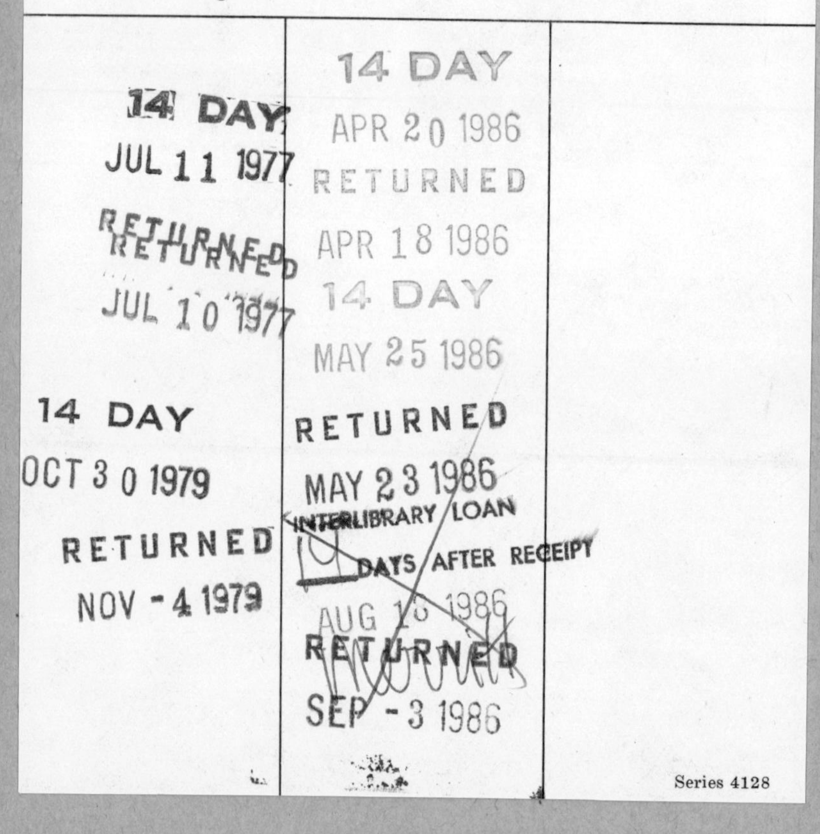
14 DAY
JUL 11 1977
RETURNED
JUL 10 1977
14 DAY
OCT 30 1979
RETURNED
NOV -4 1979
14 DAY
APR 20 1986
RETURNED
APR 18 1986
14 DAY
MAY 25 1986
RETURNED
MAY 23 1986
INTERLIBRARY LOAN
DAYS AFTER RECEIPT
RETURNED
SEP -3 1986